MICHAEL ROSEN

Many Different Kinds *of* Love

A story of life, death *and the* NHS

EBURY
PRESS

1

Ebury Press, an imprint of Ebury Publishing,
20 Vauxhall Bridge Road,
London SW1V 2SA

Ebury Press is part of the Penguin Random House group of companies
whose addresses can be found at global.penguinrandomhouse.com

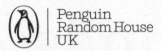

First published by Ebury Press in 2021
This edition published by Ebury Press in 2022

www.penguin.co.uk

A CIP catalogue record for this book is available from the British Library

ISBN 9781529109467

Printed and bound in Great Britain by Clays Ltd, Elcograf S.p.A.

The authorised representative in the EEA is Penguin Random House Ireland,
Morrison Chambers, 32 Nassau Street, Dublin D02 YH68

Penguin Random House is committed to a sustainable future for our
business, our readers and our planet. This book is made
from Forest Stewardship Council® certified paper.

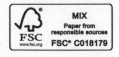

MICHAEL ROSEN is renowned for his work as a poet, performer, broadcaster and scriptwriter. He is Professor of Children's Literature at Goldsmiths, University of London and visits schools with his one-man show to enthuse children with his passion for books and poetry. In 2007 he was appointed Children's Laureate, a role which he held until 2009. While Laureate, he set up The Roald Dahl Funny Prize. He currently lives in London with his wife and children. www.michaelrosen.co.uk

For Emma

For Joe, Naomi, Eddie, Laura, Isaac, Elsie and Emile

For Dr Katie

*For all the doctors, nurses, physiotherapists,
occupational health therapists and NHS staff who
saved my life, looked after me, and helped me recover.*

Contents

Day 12. The year's seasons roll by in a night: sweats, freezes, sweats, freezes. Wondered whose mouth I had: I didn't remember it as made of sandpaper. Water is as good as ever.

Tweet from @MichaelRosenYes, 27/03/2020

i.
FEELING UNWELL

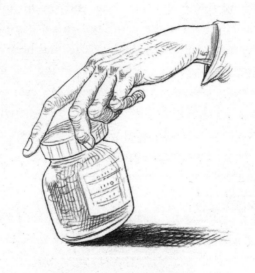

28/03/20
12:40

Hi guys,

Quick update: we've just spoken to an advanced paramedic on the phone.

He thought Mick doesn't need to go to hospital because his breathing rate is good enough and he can talk in full sentences. He thought the short breath on exertion is the effect of getting over a viral illness. (Mick has been in bed for 13 days and was getting slowly better in the last few days.)

If anything changes and the breathing rate gets more rapid, then we should call 999 – in fact he advised Michael to get to the hospital himself – I will take him of course, and not wait hours for an ambulance.

The good thing is he doesn't have a temperature and is not coughing.

What the paramedic said about getting over a viral illness is what I was thinking too, so hopefully the paramedic is absolutely right.

Take care all

Lots of love

Emma & Michael, Elsie & Emile xxxx

Get tested, says my friend John.

The GP has closed.
A recorded message at the surgery
says to not come in
and not go to A and E.
If you think you might have Covid-19,
call 111, it says.

I call 111.

I get through to the Ambulance Service
and talk to a man
who asks me some questions.
No, I'm not coughing, I say.
No, I don't feel worse today
than I felt yesterday.

He tells me to keep taking the paracetamol
and ibuprofen.

I do.

In the spare room at home
I say to Emma
it feels like I can't get enough air.
There isn't enough air.
'I can't catch up,' I say.
There are moments I feel hotter
than I've ever felt before
and moments when I am colder
than ever before.
I shudder as if I am naked
out of doors.

We look at the instructions:
Don't call the GP
Don't visit the GP
Don't go to A and E
Ring the ambulance service.
I get through.
He asks me if I'm feeling worse than yesterday.
No.
He asks me if I'm coughing.
No.
He says he thinks I'm fine.
Keep taking the paracetamol and Nurofen,

There isn't enough air.
I can't catch up.

The doorbell rings.

Emma has asked our friend, a neighbour
who is a GP, to visit.
She gives Emma
a contraption to check if
I'm absorbing oxygen and
waits outside on the doorstep.
Emma hands it back to her.
She calls out:
'You have to go to A and E right now,' she says.
'I can't really walk,' I say, 'I get the shakes
just going to the loo.'
'You have to go now,' she says, 'bump downstairs
on your bum,' she says, 'I'll ring them to tell them
you're coming,' she says.

Emma drives me to A and E
I am panting.
It's night.
The road is empty.

The moment I go in
I am surrounded with people in masks.
They put an oxygen mask over my face.

*A*fter Michael left hospital, a local GP and family friend wrote to him to describe the events of the night he was admitted. They had recently worked together on the anthology These Are the Hands: Poems from the Heart of the NHS, *giving a voice to NHS staff and raising money for NHS charities. Neither realised at the time that the staff at the heart of the NHS were about to face their hardest challenge or that Michael's life would soon depend on their care.*

12th October 2020

Dear Michael,

I know that you have been piecing together the story of your hospital admission and wanted to write to you about that evening.

As the pandemic took hold in the UK, I had seen you were unwell from your Twitter feed and said to your son Joe that I'd be happy to help.

On the day that Emma called me, a parcel arrived containing an oxygen saturation probe. Evidence was emerging of the importance of checking oxygen saturations when assessing people with COVID-19 – I had one in my doctor's bag at work, but had decided that it would be a good idea to buy one to keep at home. I did not realise at the time how important that decision and the timing of the delivery would be.

You had been feeling weak and becoming breathless. I spoke to you and Emma, checked your breathing and heart rate over the phone and said that I felt you needed to be seen and assessed. All calls were going through NHS 111 and I felt relieved to hear you were going to be checked over by a paramedic, thinking that this would be in person.

When I called back to check, Emma said a paramedic had assessed you over the phone, told her that you were likely at the tail end of the illness and advised you to stay at home unless you deteriorated. Although you had not worsened since then, I had a gut feeling at this point that I had to do something more. It sounds unscientific, but I've learnt to trust this instinct in life and in medicine.

I didn't have any PPE but decided that I needed, at the very least, to check your oxygen saturations and drove straight round. I stood at the doorway and showed Emma how to use it on my own finger and waited for her to come back.

Emma came down the stairs and said, 'It's 58'.

At first I thought this must be a mistake – that maybe she had confused this with your pulse which is also shown on the display. But when she told me that your pulse was 115, I knew there was no mistake: oxygen saturations are given as a percentage so have a maximum of 100 – a normal level is at least 95%. I had never seen an oxygen saturation this low in someone conscious.

'We need to get Michael to the hospital now,' I said, trying to remain calm and called 999. I knew that the ambulance service were overwhelmed and it would be quicker to drive you to the hospital but wasn't sure if you were going to manage getting down the stairs. While Emma and Elsie helped you down one step at a time, I continued to try and get through to the ambulance but was put on hold as the service was so busy.

With support you managed to get down the stairs, but when you got to the bottom, your legs gave way and you sank in a heap at the bottom step, resting your head on your knees. I will never forget the image of you at the bottom of the stairs, your head on your knees and your daughter Elsie gently stroking your back and whispering words of encouragement to you. I could see that you were close to collapse and gravely ill and knew I might need to step forward and try and resuscitate you without PPE. For some reason, your son Eddie* came into my mind at that point. I clearly remember thinking, 'I cannot let him die.'

A consultant at the Whittington subsequently said to me that any later would have been too late.

Emma and Elsie helped you into the car. I called ahead to A&E and spoke to a doctor to make sure they were ready for you and avoid any delays. I could see you were frightened and tried to be reassuring, saying how much better you would feel once they gave you some oxygen at the hospital. You did not have the strength to lift your head up fully or talk but gave a slight smile and a thumbs up sign before I shut the door.

Although I could see that Emma was worried, I was struck by how incredibly calmly she dealt with it all. As she drove off to the hospital, I stood at the edge of the pavement holding the oxygen probe before getting into my car. I have to admit I had a cry before pulling myself together and driving home. When I got home, my youngest daughter, Lottie ran up to me for a hug but I stopped her, realising I needed to change and shower before she touched me.

During the weeks that followed, I would speak to the doctors at the Whittington Hospital regularly. I knew the staff on ITU were rushed off their feet, so would get all the detailed medical information, updates and answers to questions and then go through them in an unrushed way with Emma. I recently found the pages of notes I made from these conversations with the incredible medical staff who were looking after you – it really brought back the rollercoaster of your journey to gradual recovery and how seriously unwell you were ...

'*getting tired on CPAP ... deteriorating ... agreed to ventilation ... ITU ... pulmonary embolism ... tinzaparin ... needing proning ... on inotropic support ... enrolled on clinical trial ... dexamethasone ... bad night ... spiking temperatures ... raised inflammatory markers ... CRP 250 ... secondary bacterial pneumonia ... responding to antibiotics ... renal and liver function improving ... taking spontaneous breaths ... tracheostomy ... weaning*

off sedation ... delirious ... for CT brain ... now off all
sedation ... calmer ... no longer needing oxygen ... transfer
for rehabilitation ... '

It really felt like a miracle when you started being able to breathe on your own again.

While you were on ITU, your poem 'These Are The Hands' became a kind of anthem for the NHS and was read on the radio, printed in newspapers and even painted onto walls. I felt profoundly moved when I heard that the staff in ITU had put it above your bed next to photos of you and your family.

Throughout all the time you were in hospital, I was constantly impressed by Emma's quiet courage and strength and her fierce protectiveness and love for you. She was always making sure that you got the best possible care and that your dignity and privacy were protected.

It was so hard for her not being able to visit you, but I remember the first time she was able to see you on a screen and her joy, that, despite all the tubes, 'He is still very much Michael'.

She showed me what quiet, real, enduring love means and how vitally important it is in these difficult times.

I am sure that, with the support of Emma and your wonderful family, you will continue to recover from this terrible illness.

With love, Katie x

* *Michael's son Eddie died of meningitis aged 18*

ii.
GOING TO HOSPITAL

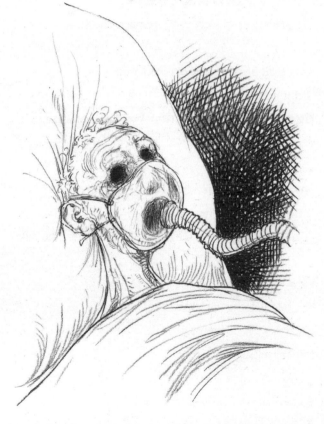

A small man comes into the ward.
He is wearing a different kind of uniform.
It's his trousers.
No one else is wearing trousers like this.
He walks up and down
with his hands behind his back.
'Breathe deeply into your masks,' he says.

Someone asks him for a bed pan.
'I don't do that,' he says.
He says that he thinks that I'm not breathing
deeply enough.

Someone asks him for a drink of water.
'I don't do that,' he says.
'You're still not breathing deeply enough,' he says.

I say that it feels as if
I'm not getting air through the mask.
I feel my chest heave.
I'm searching for air.

Someone asks him for a cup of tea.
'I don't do that,' he says.

I put my hand into the mask.
There's no air coming in.
'Excuse me,' I say,
'there's no air coming into my mask.'

He comes over.

'Your oxygen tank is empty,' he says.
'I think I need one that's full,' I say.
'Yes,' he says

Partly because I can't have any visitors
partly because my left eye doesn't work
partly because I haven't got my glasses
partly because I can't make the wifi work
partly because the wire of the charger
won't reach my bed
I can't send messages.
I feel like I'm losing home.
I can't find Emma.
I start to think she will think
that I don't want to send her messages
or talk to her.
I try to tap out a message
but I can't read it and
my thumb has hit the wrong letters.

29/03/20
22:32

Evening guys,

Just spoke to nice nurse. Michael is still on his oxygen and fluids. Also antibiotics. As I understood it, this is for the pneumonia. She said it was 'query Covid?' – they can't treat Covid with antibiotics. So will check with Dr Katie if that means Michael may not have Covid.

She said he was fine, stable, alert, awake.

I tried to find out if he was able to see his phone messages, or if anyone is able to read them to him.

Tomorrow I will contact the hospital chaplains to ask if one of them is able to visit Mick, pass on our love and maybe read some of his texts to him so that his spirits are kept up. And maybe get him some reading glasses.

STOP PRESS – Mick has just sent some texts, he said 'lovely lovely messages', 'haven't got my glasses' (!) 'very whoozy', 'pleased with breathing progress' etc.

Love to all

Emma x

I'm certain.
A certain person.
Someone who says things certainly.
It's almost an illness:
being certain, even when I'm not.
Pathologically certain, perhaps.

Now everything's not certain.
I don't know what will be.
I've got to make myself
not think that I have to be certain
about that:
listen to what the doctors say
about waiting to see what
might turn up.
Or not.

31/03/20
14:19

Hi All,

Mick has just sent me some short texts. He has eaten something and he was asking if I could send him some prunes and fruit – he said the 'geezer opposite manages to wangle it!' i.e. getting stuff sent in from outside. So this all sounds much more Mick-like!

I'm trying to see if I can send him his glasses and his fruit via a chaplain. Don't know if he will have to get a bit of spiritual guidance in exchange though ...

Love for now,

Emma

Messages from Emma to Michael

05/04/20
10:31

It's a beautiful sunny morning. Today is Sunday, day 9 – you have got yourself through 8 days and nights Mick – I know how uncomfortable and scary that has been – but you have done it – brilliant – keep calm and keep taking it v slowly. There is NO RUSH – we r not going anywhere! Xxx Love e x

Just spoke to nurse v quickly. She said you r stable, calm and just having a wash – they had to increase your levels last night by the sound of it, but it also sounds like you have settled again this morning. These nights r very hard Mick, I know. Xxx e xxx

18:52

Dr told me you are all stable again and that you look better today – that you have been in a different position on your tummy which is helping. And you've been having something to eat. This all sounds v like progress to me & I want you to be encouraged and feel reassured that although it may feel v slow going & v hard work, you r going in the right direction. Melon fruit cocktail and Tango on its way tomorrow. Lots of love e xxxx

19:58

You know the shit has hit the fan when the Queen is making a speech and it's not even Christmas … . Xxx

In the early hours of Monday 6th April a doctor rang Emma to say that they were going to re-admit Michael to intensive care and place him in an induced coma on a ventilator, and that he had agreed to this.

06/04/20
00:52
We love you so much – have a good rest now and we'll see you very soon love you xxx e xxx

A doctor is standing by my bed
asking me if I would sign a piece of paper
which would allow them to put me to sleep
and pump air into my lungs.
'Will I wake up?'
'There's a 50:50 chance.'
'If I say no?' I say.
'Zero.'
And I sign.

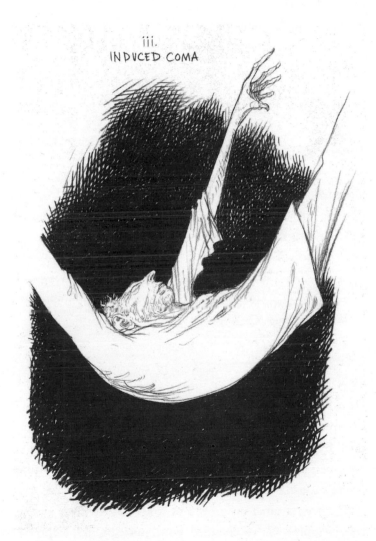

iii.
INDUCED COMA

09/04/20

Dear Michael,
We are your ITU helpers today. You are doing fantastically well and fighting hard. You still have a breathing tube, but you are doing well.
Keep fighting,
Ella C and Lizzie

10/04/20

Dear Michael,
I'm one of your helpers today and we've just given you a wash and turned you over so you don't get sore.
I'm normally a speech and language therapist working with children. I have two boys (four and two) and we sing *Bear Hunt* wherever we go. You're our hero.
Keep fighting XXX
Claire Elliott-Purdy

10/4/20 AM
Dear Michael,
It's my first night in the ITU but we are all being well looked after by the doctors and nurses. As it's my first night I've been pen pushing: recording vitals on the hour, every hour. There's a team of us making sure that your needs are met.
It's been a quiet evening, I'm told. You've been 'resting comfortably'. We've changed your position and kept you warm.

My 'day job' is a Speech and Language therapist so of course we all think you're an absolute legend. Thank you for your tireless work to foster children's love of reading!

Keep fighting Michael!

Daniel Cooper

Hi Michael,

I'm your helper this evening. Your vitals are slowly improving, including your temperature. We have wrapped you in a heated blanket and reposition you regularly to improve your lung perfusion. You're sleeping peacefully at the moment monitored and controlled by the ventilator.

We've still another eight hours together, but so far so good!

Jenny

(Physio by day, ITU helper by night!)

13/04/20–14/04/20

Dear Michael,

We have both been helping look after you this evening. The doctors have been around reviewing you a few times. We have helped reposition you and kept your medicines up-to-date.

Normally we work as physiotherapists but are finding that helping on ITU is a very rewarding experience.

We wish you all the best and keep fighting!

From Sophy and Lizzie

14/04/20

Dear Michael,
My name is Aime, and I am one of the nurses here in ITU. You were admitted in the early hours of 5 April and immediately intubated. That means that a tube was placed in your throat to help you breathe. You were very sick when you came in and over the next few days you were proned (turned on your front) for long periods of time, this is to help with your oxygen. You have been kept fully sedated to allow you to tolerate the tube and to give your lungs and other organs time to recover. We were very worried about you for a number of days but I'm glad to see that now you are starting to improve and you are receiving a lot less support from the ventilator. You still have some way to go until you recover, but your body is now fighting this virus and I promise we will keep giving you the best care we can give, until we get you back on your feet.

Best wishes,
Aime

14/04/20

Dear Michael,
Holly, Emma and Ally have been looking after you today.

As today has turned into this evening you have looked so much more relaxed and comfortable, which is just fantastic. We've done our best to keep you clean, warm and comfortable today.

We hope you get some rest this evening and we look forward to seeing you in improved health tomorrow.

Just. Keep. Going.

Thursday 16/04/20

Dear Michael,
My name is Heloise and I have been looking after you today. I have been helping the nurses in intensive care, but usually work as a speech and language therapist (storytelling with toddlers). I first met you the first time you came into this intensive care ward: it was on Sunday 29th March, the day the clocks changed (and I had had a lot of trouble with my digital fidgetal botch that morning!).

I hope to see you soon and I hope very much that you carry on improving!

Thank you for the books.

Best wishes,

Heloise

Dear Michael,
Today is Thursday 16th April, Captain Tom Moore has just finished his hundredth lap around his garden and raised £12,000,000 for the NHS! What a feat!

I'm usually a physio but helping out this evening to keep up with notes and whatever odd jobs are needed.

You are looking well and comfortable today, the doctors have said you're doing great. Keep going! Looking forward to seeing you when you open your eyes.

Best wishes,

Claire

Dear Michael,

My name is Beth and I have been the nurse looking after you overnight (Thursday 16th). I normally work at Great Ormond Street Hospital looking after children but have been moved here to help look after adults (I call you guys big children).

You have done really well overnight. You are starting to move little bits which is excellent. Hope you continue this great progress. You've got this!! Looking forward to meeting you when you wake up, you read my favourite book … *We're Going On a Bear Hunt*.

All the best,

Beth

Dear Michael,

My name is Margie, I'm one of the nurses who admitted you in the ICU on 29/03/20. At that time you only required a CPAP Machine which helped you and we were able to move you back to the ward.

On your second ICU admission, you required a ventilator to take over your breathing due to your further deterioration. You required quite a lot of ventilator support, the ICU team had to prone you, meaning you had to lie on your belly to improve your oxygenation. This procedure required seven people to reposition you carefully.

The ICU team was so glad to see you improving every day. Your breathing is much better compared to previous days. You are now breathing with less support from the ventilator. Your vital signs are stable also. We are hoping to see you improving every day. Take one day at a time. You will get there soon.

All the best Michael!

Margie

(ICU nurse)

18/04/20–19/04/20

Dear Michael,

My name is Natasha. I'm usually employed in the community but because the school I work in is closed, I'm helping out in ICU.

I'm helping Diane (staff nurse) to look after you and Elaine (a physio) is also on the team tonight.

This evening one of the IV lines in your neck was taken out because the doctors were happy with your progress. You've also been moving your arms about a little and I think you might have been aware of us speaking to you.

You still have a tube in to help you breathe but you're taking your own breaths and your blood oxygen levels have remained pretty stable. Keep fighting Michael – the children (and adults) need to hear more of your wonderful poems and stories. Thank you for all you've written so far.

20/04/20

Dear Michael,

My name is Sara. I'm helping to look after you with Sheeba (urology nurse) and Raquel (infection control nurse) today.

I normally work as a dental hygienist and therapist in the community but I'm helping out in ITU due to COVID-19. All the doctors and nurses are happy with your progress!

We have all worked together to keep you warm and comfortable today.

Thank you for all your poems and books you have written, especially the 60th anniversary of the NHS poem, it is beautiful.

I hope you continue to improve!

Keep fighting!

Sara

23/04/20–24/04/20

Hello Michael!

I am looking after you today with Kazia (a nurse from GOSH – she's wonderful!).

I've been asking you to blink and squeeze my hand to communicate and you have been diligently obliging.

You're doing great. The doctors are keeping an eye on your blood pressure.

Your NHS 60 years anniversary poem is touching to all working here in ICU – thank you. Please send it to Boris Johnson!!

I really hope you recover well.

Best of luck,

Kajal Doshi (physio/ ICU helper)

26/04/20
Day shift

Hey Michael,

My name is Alison and I am the helper looking after you today with Sarah, who is your nurse.

I am a physiotherapist normally, but have been redeployed with a lot of my colleagues, many who have helped care for you.

I also have a two-year-old girl who I often hear 'going on a bear hunt' and when we need to get her walking we say 'it's a bear!' which gets her running, so thank you very much, it helps our walks.

Today has been a busy day for you, lots of doctors and nurses have been caring for you, you have been well cared for. You have been restless at times but I have been there to hold your hand.

You have been for a CT scan today, which keeps all the nurses and doctors on their toes! Your poem for the 60th anniversary of the NHS is very fitting at the moment. Keep fighting and getting better.

Alison

28/04/20
08:30

Good morning Michael,
It's a pleasure to look after you. I am Pat, a lung nurse specialist currently working in ITU to help the wonderful ITU nurses look after you.

It's lovely to see all the photos of your family smiling and showing how much you are loved.

We will keep you comfortable, and talk to you all through the shift to let you know what we're doing.

My kids were brought up on your poems and loved them.

We have given you a lovely wash and brushed your thick hair.

At 13:30 hours:
Michael started blinking his eyes, moved both arms and legs. He squeezed the doctor's/consultant's hand to respond to her questions.

Michael confirmed that he was uncomfortable, he was repositioned and given some pain relief.

29/04/20
Good afternoon Michael,
It's Claire the physio again! You must be sick of me talking to you today, we've been chatting a lot to keep you stimulated so your blood pressure rises. We've also been playing some

of your stories on a laptop, I love the way you tell them, you're so animated!

You're turning your head when I'm talking to you as well! Great stuff!

Every time I see you, you look a little better Michael which is lovely to see.

Keep going!! You've got this!

Claire

Night shift

Hi Michael,

My name is Lizzie and I am your helper tonight. I'm normally a physio working in outpatients but I'm currently helping out in ITU during the Covid pandemic.

I looked after you on one of your first nights, so it's so lovely to see how far you've come. You still have a breathing tube going into your throat, meaning you aren't able to speak. So unfortunately for you it's mostly me chatting away to you! I seemed to get a response when I mentioned that you supported Arsenal judging from your pictures, but you didn't seem impressed when I told you I was a Derby County fan!

You are currently sleeping very peacefully and look very comfortable.

Thank you for all the lovely books and poems you have gifted us, *We're Going On A Bear Hunt* is one of my favourite childhood books! We have also laminated the poem you did for the NHS anniversary which is by your bed.

Keep going, keep fighting and keep being so strong.
Lizzie xx (physio)

02/05/20–03/05/20
Hi again Michael. It's Natasha again! I worked with you a couple of weeks ago and it's wonderful to see how much better you are looking! You're trying to communicate now by mouthing words and nodding or shaking your head or using facial expressions.

At the moment, you have some padded mitten type-things on your hands. This is just to stop you from accidentally pulling out any tubes, like your tracheostomy tube which connects to the ventilator, or the NG tube in your nose which carries nutrition and hydration to your stomach.

Your blood pressure has been fluctuating a bit – it is sometimes on the low side so we have to keep waking you up regularly to stimulate you and bring it back up. Sorry if this has been annoying!

Your nurse this shift has been Sara, who is wonderful, and your main helper has been Sophie, who is a physio. We are rooting for you!

Overnight
Good morning Michael,

My name is Sara, I'm one of the ITU nurses looking after you overnight with the much appreciated help of Dennis, one of the other ITU nurses.

You've much improved over the past week although you have kept us quite busy overnight! Your blood pressure decided that it fancied being a yo-yo and we've had to do a good amount of deep suctioning via your trachy (the breathing tube in your throat which helps the gas exchange of oxygen and carbon dioxide in your lungs). I'm really sorry this is so unpleasant – it's so important to get that mucus out of your lungs.

I'm sorry I can't write more, with the pandemic each nurse has multiple patients – but keep fighting! You'll go home soon.

Sara

02/05/20
18:07

Hi All,
Mick is experiencing delirium at the moment and this is making him quite agitated, hallucinating and moving his arms and legs around.

This is very common when someone has been sedated for so long and also when they have pneumonia, etc. They are adjusting his medication, trying small doses of different drugs to try to help this because they can't begin to wean him from the ventilator until he is more calm, as he risks pulling out vital tubes.

But, delirium is not permanent, and although it may take some days, if not longer with Mick, it should pass.

He is now on the next lot of antibiotics for the pneumonia as advised by the microbiologist.

The doctor asked me for some music last evening and apparently some Django Reinhardt seemed to soothe him a bit!

Elsie and I made a playlist for him this morning which is now taped up on the wall by his bed and the staff have already played him some of the tracks!

Love to all
Emma x

04/05/20
13:45

Hi Michael,
My name is Holly. I am currently helping nurse Jo in looking after you. It's so lovely to see how well you are progressing. Every time I come into work you are getting stronger and starting to reduce the use of the ventilator.

Today I have made you a YouTube playlist of all the songs your family sent us. Some absolute tunes on there. You have been listening to the playlist all day. I think I am enjoying it as much as you.

We are going to video call your family shortly. It's always important for recovery to hear familiar voices – keep fighting, I know you can do this.

Best wishes,
Holly

May the fourth be with you!
Dear Michael,
My name is Joe Lynch, an ex-ITU nurse who answered the call to help with the influx of COVID-19 patients in the intensive care. I am writing in retrospect as I have looked after you twice so far. About five weeks ago and also last week. It is amazing to see how far you have come. I was the nurse who shaved you just before a video call with your wife. Sorry to have you clean shaven but you can only imagine how curly your beard had got.

The second time I looked after you I spoke to you a lot.

You seemed quite agitated and I know this is such a confusing time for you, I am truly sorry. Everybody says hello to you every day as you have been with us for 29 days. Everyone knows you and is rooting for you to keep improving and getting stronger.

Things may seem like a dream when you are here. You may remember vivid memories or images, sounds or even smells. That is very normal. Your family have been sending their love every day.

All the best in your recovery,

Joe (nurse)

06/05/20
16:30

Afternoon Michael,

It's Holly (helper) again. Today I am looking after you with lovely nurse Joy.

We have had a busy day so far. It started off with spa time – a bed bath, hair comb, nail cut and clean and we also shaved your beard. Sorry, we know you usually have a beard, that's just so we can keep the area around your trachy (the place where the tube sits in your neck) clean. We have placed some pads on your eyes to keep them closed as they had been open and you need some rest.

We then spent some time listening to your fab playlist again. You appear much more comfortable and settled today. You have been breathing with the ventilator today and your oxygen requirement has been reduced, all great progressions.

We are going to let you rest now as we have moved you to a new bed, I hope it's comfortable.

I'm unsure whether I will work with you again Michael as the ITU unit is slowly returning to normal. This means 'helpers' will go back to our usual jobs. I should be heading back to my bladder and bowel team. I wish you all the best with your recovery. You are a fighter and can do this.

Best wishes,

Holly

PS Happy Birthday for tomorrow

07/05/20

Dear Michael,

HAPPY BIRTHDAY!

It's been so lovely to help look after you today on your birthday! You've been a popular chap today – FaceTime calls from your family and a birthday card!

You were also treated to a rendition of Happy Birthday from about 15 ICU staff around your bedside and a round of applause from staff and one of the other patients!

You continue to improve and I know how proud everyone is of you.

Monique is the ITU nurse who is looking after you today, along with help from Bruce and Dennis – they've all taken fantastic care of you.

I wish you all the best in your recovery – get well soon!

Sophy (physiotherapist)

Monique (ITU nurse)

15/05/20
14:43

Hi All,

Some small steps of improvement: the agitation and delirium seem to have lifted. Mick has been calmer, more settled and has been off all sedation for the last few days. He is responding to some commands with hand squeezing, arm movements etc., and has some improved function in his muscles which are obviously very weakened after so long.

They think he may have some nerve damage and I don't know if this could be permanent or temporary and what the cause is, but they can't do an MRI scan of the brain until he is off the ventilator. The two scans of his head that they did do in the past couple of weeks have both shown nothing. He is still on the antibiotics for the cavitating pneumonia but his markers for infection have come down.

I asked about his Covid status. As of 27th April he was positive and they won't do another test until the end of this month.

The doctors have been making progress with weaning him from the ventilator by doing breathing trials, following the plan made by the Respiratory Physios. He was on an oxygen mask (i.e. not the ventilator!) for an hour and a half yesterday and today he has done 4 hours this morning and the plan is for 4 hours this afternoon. I think this is a real improvement and I hope that his responses will continue to improve slowly as all the drugs gradually leave his system.

All love for now

Emma x

15/05/20
Night shift

Hi Michael,

My name is Carmen and I have been your nurse looking after you for the past two nights.

I originally admitted you to the intensive care unit 40 days ago during the night when you were having some difficulty in breathing and showing symptoms of virus.

Well what a rollercoaster you have been on since then!! And you are still here to tell the tale.

Today was a good day for you, you managed to breathe on your own with just the tracheostomy mask twice during the day, four hours at a time.

Overnight I am putting you back on the ventilator to let you rest and give you the strength to breathe on your own for even longer tomorrow.

The physios have drafted a tracheostomy weaning plan with the aim of helping you to breathe on your own again and getting you out onto a regular ward where you can spend a little bit more time recovering.

I have really noticed your level of cognition has started to return and you now answer my questions with nodding or shaking your head which is really nice to see.

I have read some of your birthday cards and messages to tonight and continually remind you where you are, which seems to help when you start to get a bit agitated.

I have done lots of suctioning of your airway as there are still lots of secretions but not as much as the previous nights so you are making progress!

Keep strong and remember – little steps in the right direction!

Get well soon,

Carmen

16/05/20
Nightshift

Dear Michael,

It's Natasha again, one of the helpers on ITU (usually I'm a speech and language therapist). It's been brilliant to see how much better you are since the last time I helped to look after you.

Although you can't voice yet because of the cuffed tracheostomy tube (which means that no air reaches your vocal cords) you have been able to indicate yes/no and with a combination of some guess work and your expressive non-verbal communication skills you are able to ask some questions/make comments. You have had quite a lot of secretions still and you have needed a lot of suctioning which has meant you haven't had as much rest as you might like.

Tomorrow, I am told, they want to try you off the respirator completely. I am crossing my fingers that you will manage as this would be a huge step forward in your recovery.

There have been moments when you have been distressed and needed lots of reassurance. This is completely understandable. Being in ITU under the current circumstances can be incredibly disorientating and traumatic.

My hope is that you will get lots of hugs and love from your family to make up for all this time you have been apart, once you are free to go home.

I'm not sure if I'll be back again next week and if I am I hope that you will be on a ward rather than here and that much closer to going home – although I will of course miss working with you!

It has been a true honour. As I mentioned before, my two children love your poems and books and it has been a privilege to help in looking after you.

Good luck for tomorrow and I wish you safely home soon.

Natasha

17/05/20

It's Claire the physio … again.

I haven't looked after you for a while, you've progressed so much since I last saw you, you are squeezing our hands and wiggling your toes when asked. Today we went up to the fourth floor and met your lovely wife Emma and looked out over London. It was really special to see you with your family. You are now resting in bed listening to your playlist which I am also really enjoying! I used to listen to Dave Brubeck's quartet with my mum – and tried to learn the saxophone and failed miserably.

KEEP GOING!

Claire

17/05/20
18:10

Hi All,

At short notice today, the hospital allowed me to visit Mick. They wheeled his bed out onto the 4th Floor where there is a great view of London so I could sit with him. I played him all the little messages twice and he definitely responded to them.

He is off the ventilator and was on a low level of oxygen (28%) and they hope they will be able to step him down to the ward (high dependency) soon. They've got a programme of music, TV and radio worked out for him to help him reconnect with his surroundings, and I handed over the iPad.

He has now also had a negative Covid test. Bloody hurrah!

All love

Emma x

17/05/20–18/05/20
Overnight

Hi Michael,

Your nurse Ash and I have been looking after you this evening.

You've been coughing quite a bit, bringing up a lot of phlegm – that meant we haven't had to suction you as much – every cloud …

The coughing has made it hard for you to sleep but you have gotten a couple of hours of shut eye.

Communication has been very challenging for you this evening/morning. You've been trying to tell us a few things but we haven't been able to understand – and that's been very frustrating for you. But you've told us you're comfortable and you've stayed positive in spite of it all.

Keep fighting – it will all be worth it.

Dan, SLT/helper

19/05/20
Night shift

Hi Michael,

My name is Ellen, your night nurse. I've looked after you before (maybe two weeks ago) but didn't have the chance to write in this diary. You still have the tracheostomy but you're not needing the breathing machine any more. A scan of your chest was also done during the day and it has shown improvement of your lungs. The doctors are happy for you to be transferred to a 'normal' ward later in the day. Also, your swabs came back as Covid negative.

Wishing you a speedy recovery,

Ellen

19/05/20
Day 43

Hi Michael!

My name is Wincey, one of the nurses here in the intensive care unit.

I have looked after you several times on your early days here in the unit when you were critically unwell.

I didn't manage to write on those specific days for there were loads of nursing interventions needing to be done for you.

I am so happy and pleased to see how you are recovering so well! You've been through a lot and your journey with this pandemic was not an easy one yet your progress is remarkable.

Please be patient with yourself. Slowly but surely! I can't blame you that you really wanted to go home – hospital can be quite boring at times!

You celebrated your birthday with us. I wished for your speedy recovery, I am pretty sure your family misses you a lot and they are thinking about you every single minute of every day!

I cannot wait to the day you will go home and be reunited with your family. I am sure it will be full of joy, laughter and overflowing with love and gratitude. You will not fully remember all the events that have happened but it is expected as you received so many sedatives in the early stages of your admission here on the unit.

You take good care Michael and it has been a privilege to have looked after you!

May you continue to touch and inspire every human being you will encounter! God bless.

Your nurse – Wincey

20/05/20

Dear Michael,

I'm Ewa – one of the physiotherapists working in ITU.

Yesterday we used the speaking valve on your tracheostomy for the first time and we could hear your voice to the first time – very exciting we did!!! Today, you sat out in the chair and are due to go to meet up with your family. You are making good progress every day. I can't wait to see you stand up and walk.

Keep going and stay strong.

All the best,

Ewa

21/05/20
Night shift

Dear Michael,

My name is Louise, I am one of the sisters here on intensive care.

It was so nice to hear that today you had your tracheostomy removed and you are now breathing unaided, with just a small amount of extra oxygen.

Talking to you this evening, you are expressing how you have had to relearn many things as you recover from your illness. This is true, but remember to give yourself the time to do this, you will get stronger day by day, be patient if you can. We will help you all we can to rebuild your strength and support you as you continue on your journey of recovery.

So pleased to be able to talk with you, hear your voice.

Best wishes,

Louise

22/05/20
18:08

Hi All,

I'm very happy to say that Michael is moving out of ICU tonight and will be going to Meyrick Ward.

He has no tracheostomy tube and no oxygen support apart from a nebulizer. He is talking, still confused (delirium) at times and is trying to piece it all together obviously, but slowly becoming more Mick-like.

I'm going to the hospital in a bit to deliver him some comfy bed clothes, a soft blanket, his own toiletries etc. for when he is able to move a bit more and get out of bed.

He will have been in hospital 8 weeks tomorrow and has spent 47 days in ICU.

Looking forward to a glass of wine later!

Love to all

Emma x

iv.
RECOVERY

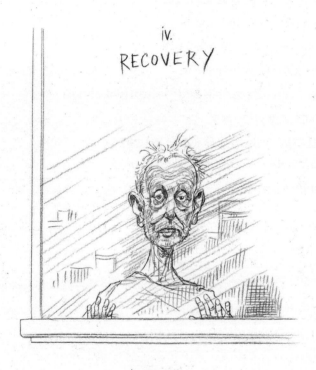

PART ONE

Very poorly.

It's something they say about me.

Every so often a doctor or nurse

stands by my bed and says,

'You were very poorly.'

I'm starting to expect it.

They often seem pleased – surprised almost –

that I'm less poorly.

I get the feeling that some people

who were very poorly, died.

I didn't die.

I'm wearing mittens.
Why am I wearing mittens?
They are dark blue, puffy and tied tightly
round my wrists.
I try to rip them off
but a hand in a padded mitten
is no good at untying the laces
that hold them on.

I try tearing at it with my teeth.
The night nurse comes over.
and asks me why am I trying to take my mittens off?
I say that it's because I don't want them
and I can't sleep with them on.
She says, Relax, lie back and
save your energy.

She says the word 'Energy'
like a Tai Chi teacher,
as if it is something sacred.

'Save your en-er-gy,' she says again.
'Lie down and move up the bed,' she says
'your feet are touching the end of the bed.'

I say, 'My feet are touching the end of the bed
because the bed is too small.'
'Relax,' she says,
'save your en-er-gy.'

I put my head on the pillow
and feel the drumming of a washing machine
from somewhere below
as if it runs up through the backbone of the building.
I see it churning the sheets and gowns
blankets and pyjamas of us all
boiling them clean and stiff.

Perhaps there are pressers down there too,
that flatten them like blocks of paper,
sometimes so thin
the poppers don't close.

I turn over on to the ear that doesn't work
to see if the working ear can pick up
the washing machine.
There's no sound
but the rhythm, the skeleton of sound
reaches me somehow.

I think it's the middle of the night.

There must be people down there
feeding the machines.

They say they're weaning me.
I remember weaning:
weaning our babies.
Or were they toddlers by then?
Teaching them that there's this stuff
called food.
Now they're weaning me.
I think they're weaning me on to breathing air.
Coming off the stuff that comes through machines.
They're keen on weaning.
They keep saying it.
We're weaning you, they say.

A doctor asks me whether I've had
hallucinations or nightmares
or terrifying delirium.
I say no.

She says that they are getting reports
that people who've been in intensive care
are experiencing this
and they're troubled by it,
are you?
I say no

She says, We gave you a lot of
mind-changing drugs, so we wouldn't be surprised
if you said you were suffering from this.
Were you upset or agitated by anything like this?

I said that I dream 'The Christmas Carol'
and write a new version in my head
then become distressed that I can't write it down.
Mmmm, she says.

I also keep dreaming of a German Christmas party.
It's always the same part.
I've never been to a German Christmas party

but I'm sitting outside at night in a garden
wrapped in blankets
and I know that I can't move my legs.
My legs won't move.
Someone explains that they throw purple berries
into the air.
They do it:
they throw the berries in the air,
and the berries burst with a flash
like little stars
and everyone cheers.
They tell me the word for the purple berries
is 'Wassbeeren'.
Again the berries burst in the night sky
and everyone cheers.
I have that dream again and again, I say.
'Mmm,' she says, 'Nothing terrifying?'

I'm disturbed by another dream.
I imagine that just before I got ill
I came across a statement, a kind of manifesto
from a German farmer.
It was a reply to the hate coming from
neo-Nazis in his neighbourhood.
He comes towards me

wearing a stone-washed bib-and-brace.
He stands alongside his 1950s tractor
with his family around him.
His manifesto tells how we can only
go on if we love each other,
we have to find many different kinds of love
he says, love for lovers, love for our children
love for our colleagues, love even for people
we don't know.
If we don't, we will destroy ourselves.

What makes me sad about this dream
Is that I keep getting to the point
where I am thinking:
Where is this manifesto?
Who is the farmer?
I feel sure he gave it to me before I got ill.
How did I get to meet him and his family?
Where was it?
And then it goes.

It's not nightmarish.
More a matter of regret
that I've lost track of something.

A nurse tells me every day
that Emma has rung
and that they are telling her everything.
I think of the space between
here and home where Emma is.
It's only a few streets but
it's a gulf.
In that world I used to get up
and make myself breakfast.
I'd sit down with Emma and plan
what I would do over the next few months.
Here I wait for a meal
and I'm asked if I've opened my bowels:
Was it a big one, a medium one or a small one?
I am ticked off if I lie too far from the centre
    of the bed.
A nurse walks past singing
'No woman no cry'.

It's four in the morning.
The nurse tells me she is
doing my 'obs':
blood pressure, oxygen level,
temperature,
and what she picks up
from looking at me for 30 seconds.

I offer up my arm for the pressure sleeve,
my finger for the oxygen clip,
my ear for the temperature.
I wait while she looks at me.

She writes down the figures.
There is now a ledger telling
the story of all my ups and downs.
I have become an account.

I turn on the bed and
into the pillow.
They don't belong to me.

My body has become theirs.
They have it.

They tell me about my liver,
my kidneys, my lungs, my heart.
It's all in the account.

I move my hand over my chest.
There's nothing else to do.
My ribs stand out like the ridges
on our griddle.
Moobs have mostly gone.
My finger follows my sternum down:
a bump.
That's not been there before, surely.
A hard bony bump between the sternum
and one of the ribs.
It's a new friend.

I feel my thumb joint.
The mildly arthritic one.
It's only a bother when my son
grabs it when we're wrestling.
Is it bigger?
I don't think so.
Are arthritic bumps
anywhere else?

I explore my bones.
I run my fingers over joints
the back of my neck,
down to my ankles and toes.
Nothing bumpy.

Then I remember
I'm getting sore at the top
of my bum-crease.
A bed-sore person came round
the other day and got us all rolling over
to one side so that he could inspect us
and he found, he said, a redness,
down there.
Lie more on your side, he said,
so you share the bits of you that
take your weight in the bed.
I handed him my little tub of Vaseline
and he smeared it on.

I feel down there.
My finger finds a bump.
The tailbone that is usually
a snug fit at the bottom of my spine
curling under my bum
is now like the root vegetables
that people put on the internet
decorated with suggestive lumps.
The lump runs under my left buttock
so when I sit on my tailbone
it pinches the top of my bum-crease.
I have two new friends.

It's night.
I press the button
on the buzzer strung up by my bed
to call for the nurse.
I want the bed pan.
I can't walk
but I can lift myself up enough
to squat on a bed pan.
I call for the nurse.
It's night.

I call for the nurse
but she doesn't come.
I press the buzzer again.
I am sweating.
It's night.

I call out.
I shout.
I am sorry that I am waking people up.
I press the buzzer.
It's night.

I soil myself
and feel ashamed.

I long to be home
where I could perhaps have
crawled to the loo, I think.

The nurse comes.
I say that I'm sorry, very sorry
that I have soiled myself.
She says sorry
she was dealing with another patient.
I think: rows and rows of beds
like soldiers in the First World War
and here she is struggling to get round
and I've gone and soiled myself.
And she is a woman I've never met
who has never met me
who has to clean me up.

I am sorry, very sorry.
She says that I shouldn't worry.
She slips away in the dark.
It's night.

Two people come to my bed
and say they are physios.
They say that I need to get moving.
They try to get me to stand up
but I can't.
When I try to make my legs support me
nothing works.
They stand on either side of me
and prop me up.
The whole of my body is shaking.
I look down at my legs.
They are shrunken, white and wrinkled.
They look like my father's legs
when he was dying.
I'm panting. Gasping.
Can I lie down? I say.
They say they will come again soon.

A few days later
a woman comes who says she is a physio.
She says she will help me sit
on the edge of the bed.
She props me up and says
'Sit up as straight as you can
and clench your bum.'
I try to but I am shaking and gasping

and fall back into the bed.

A few days later, two guys from Liverpool
turn up by the side of my bed.
They say they're going to get me to walk.
They lever me out of the bed,
prop me up and say,
'See if you can take a step.'

I can't.

They seem disappointed.
I am gasping
and they look at me surprised by the
rasping noise I'm making.
They put me back to bed.
They say they will be back soon.

As I lie in bed
I remember that they all said
that it's a good exercise for someone
lying in bed to lift your leg
and hold it in the air for a count of ten,
I think they all said that.

Sometimes I try to do that.

One day
they bring a hydraulic hoist to my bed
put me in a sling,
lift me into a chair
and wheel me to a window
on the fourth floor that looks out over London.
Emma is there and the children.
We sit with our masks on.
I have a blanket.
We are together.
I feel bad that I am so helpless.
That I can't move.

I start to feel weak and dizzy.
They wheel me away
and I can't look round to wave goodbye.

I've forgotten my shoes.
I don't know what my shoes were.
I try to remember my feet in shoes.
The only shoes I know
are the ones I have here:
black plastic crocs.
But what shoes did I used to wear?
I've forgotten my shoes.

At school
we made brown paint.
We mixed black and red.
This made brown.

My brain
makes a view.
It mixes left eye fog
with right eye clear.
This makes blur.

I keep making a plan
to have a writers' cricket match.
I see myself sitting with the poet John Agard.
He shows me how he spins the ball.
We sit together,
he raises his hand
and carves a line through the air.

'John,' I say, 'what did Michael Holding
call that fast ball that cut back?'
'The Doctor,' he says,
'he served up treatment to stop
the batsman scoring.'
He laughs.
It fades.

A few days later
it comes back.
The same plan: a writers' cricket match
that never takes place,
John flicking his fingers,
carving a line through the air.
'What did Michael Holding call that fast ball
that cut back?' I say.
'The Doctor,' he says and laughs.
It fades.

A doctor stands by my bed
and says that I have three blood clots
in my lungs.
I picture three reddish brown scabs
stuck in the passage-ways of my lungs,
nestling in the alveoli:
little bubble-like cul-de-sacs
that I drew for my Biology exam
when I was 16.

She says, 'Blood clots are always a worry
because they can get into the blood stream
and cause heart attacks and strokes.'
I see the scabs heading downstream in my veins
getting stuck in the heart I dissected for
Biology
or pushing into my brain and killing off
a chunk of that cauliflower-looking thing.
'How worried should I be?' I say.
'You'll probably digest them,' she says.

I remember picking scabs off my knee
on camping holidays
and eating them.
I must have digested them.

The nights are long and sad.
I feel like I don't sleep at all
and lie in the dark
listening to the monitors and drips.
Different parts of our bodies
turned into numbers and beeps.

Someone behind a curtain
is talking on the phone.
There are sirens.
A nurse says she is going to do my blood pressure
and wraps my arm in an inflatable sleeve.
'It's very low,' she says.
'you need to keep drinking.
And move your arms.'
I drink some water
and wave my arms in the air.
The nurse asks me to hold a strip of paper
under my tongue.
'It'll tell me what your temperature is,' she says.
'Don't chew it,' she says.
'I'm not chewing it,' I say.
She goes.
The nights are long and sad.

Dream

I'm in a town
and I ask someone the way.
He says, you keep straight on
till you get to the desert.
Don't cross the desert.
Go round it.

I make an effort to remember
what he said:
Don't cross the desert
Go round it.

I think of those two men
who tried to walk across Australia
but didn't make it.

I chew over the word 'liminal'
and remember how in the class I teach
at university we talked about how portals
in fantasy stories are 'liminal',
a space or moment 'in between worlds'
or on the edge of one world but not quite
in another,
where things are transient, temporary
or provisional
but it can be a moment full of promise
or it can be a moment of anxiety or danger:
think the Alice books,
Alice going down the rabbit hole,
and through a looking glass.
Or sitting in the waiting area at an airport.
I think of a train journey to a summer camping
    holiday
when I was 8 years old, with the land one side
and the sea on the other.

I start to believe the edges of my body are liminal,
they are touching other worlds
sheets, blankets, the bed, the 'fence'
on the side of the bed, the pillows
and it is all this that stops me sleeping:

they are all edges.
So I bring my hand up to my face
and put it under my cheek.
It feels like I've found myself
something that's not on an edge
and I'm back with me.

I sleep well that night.

Fumbling the phone.
Shut the foggy eye.
Thumbs miss the keys.
Trying to get through to you.
Type rubbish.
Hope you don't think that
I don't care enough to write
to you properly.
Nothing comes out right.
Dizzy. Even in bed.
Even lying down, dizzy.

We get FaceTime to work
and there she is on my phone
telling me that I'm going to be OK
and she is thinking of me
and wants me to get better
and I see my own shrunken moon look
and raggedy hair
on the phone screen alongside her
lovely face
but we've connected.
There's a bridge we can see each other on.

You've given me an iPad
and I'm trying to use it.
You say I should stroke it
with my hand.
Upwards.
Or sideways.
I can't see it properly because
one of my eyes doesn't work.
A nurse takes it off me
and gets it to play
'Under Milk Wood'.

You've put that on there for me.
I listen
and think again how beautiful it is
how full of life and sadness
and love
how we watched a filmed version of it
together
and how we loved it
and I wish that I could write as well as that
and that voices could read what I wrote
with such feeling

with such a sense of a place and a time
but then I think
what matters now
is that I can listen to it.

Emma sends in a furry blanket
and a duvet that has a black and white checked cover.
At last
my hands and feet are warm.
I put my cheek next to the fur
or the linen of the duvet cover.
I feel safe
and strong.
Emma is with me here.

My feet are a long way off.
When I look at them with my good eye
I can see the nails are starting to look like
animal claws.
The nurses say that they are not allowed
to cut them.
At night I feel a nail cutting into the toe
beside it.
And another.
And another.
The nails scrape the blanket over my feet
and I can't think how to reach them
and clip them.
Are the nurses allowed to use clippers on them?
No.

I stare.
'My eyes are different,' I say,
'my right eye is the same as it was,
but my left eye is blurred,' I say.
No one knows why.
I cover up first one eye
and then the other.
The right eye is clear.
The left eye is trying to see through
something.
It could almost be
that a plastic sheet has got stuck
inside the eye.
I tell everyone who comes to see me.
No one knows why this has happened.

I have an idea:
I call Emma late at night
and ask her to come and get me.
'Can you tell them I want to come home tonight?'
   I say.
'I can come back to the hospital the following day,'
   I say
'I can't cope with the nights anymore.'

She reminds me that I can't walk
I can't even stand up.
'You need to stay there a little bit longer,' she says.
I realise she's right
but it feels such a shame.
I had told myself a story
of us cuddling up together
or sleeping peacefully in our bed
having breakfast together
and just popping back to the hospital
for my jabs and pills.
But it was just that: a story.
There are more days
and more nights to come.

The ward is dark.
I can hear a metal purr
from the other side,
then a bubbling syrup.
He coughs.
More bubbling.
It must be coming up from his chest.
The metal purr must be sucking it up.
A light is on behind the curtains
over there.
The nurse tells him to keep still.

I'm growing sand on my skin.

I brush my hand over my shoulders.

They're sandy.

I brush the sand away.

A few days later:

more sand.

No pain.

No soreness.

No rash.

Just sand.

I'm growing sand.

Mothers
with their new born babies
were confined.
I recall 'confinement':
someone in an old novel I read
long ago
was confined.
Perhaps in its own way
it was good:
you didn't have to do
usual work –
plenty of work coping with this new event though.
People helped you,
you had time to wonder
between feeds;
let your body
become what it could:
millions of cells
growing, grouping.
And yet:
a barrier between here
and out there.
Others in charge.

There was an advert in Underground stations
when I was a child.
Two small children
who we see from behind
walking along a long empty road
holding hands,
dark trees on either side.

The ad line was:
'Children's shoes have far to go.'

I used to feel sad for the children:
so alone
so far from home.

I see the ad
again and again.

You sent in giant yellow sultanas.
You know me.

Every morning
I drop them into the porridge
that the nurses bring us.

As I sip
I discover the sultanas
basking in the deep,
swelling in the hot milk
and I nibble them
one by one
with my front teeth
pushing my tongue
against the wrinkles
and flesh.

I have a tube sticking up my nose.
Or out of my nose.
I don't know why I have a tube
sticking up my nose.
Or out of my nose.
It's there all the time.
It's been there for as long as I remember.
I feel it rest on my neck:
rubbery and clammy.
It could be a worm.
Or a slug.

One night it falls out.
I call the nurse.
I say, the tube has fallen out of my nose.
She seems cross.
She asks me why I pulled the tube out of my nose.
I say, I didn't pull it out of my nose,
it came out.
She says that she'll have to put it back.

She collects together some instruments,
pulls the curtain round the bed
and shines the light on me.
I hear her breathing next to me.

Then I feel the worm going up my nose
A moment later I feel it going down my throat.
I gag.
The worm keeps on going.

The nurse turns off the light
and takes the instruments away.

In the morning
The doctor comes round
And says it's time to take the tube out.
We'll do that today, he says.
You're doing very well, he says.
You were very poorly.

Emma says that I'm going to a
Rehabilitation hospital in St Pancras.
She says she's seen pictures of it,
people sitting in a garden,
a gym,
and she's read a statement
about getting people back on their feet.

It feels like a way out,
A route to getting better.
I see myself sitting in a garden
in a wheelchair with a blanket over me
looking at the trees.
I imagine me standing up
and walking across the grass.
I am sure it's going to be good.

V.
REHAB

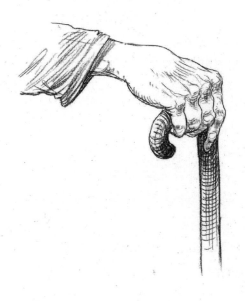

What did I do all day
after I came out of intensive care?
How did I spend the day?
How did I fill those hours?
No reading, no radio, no TV
no internet, no conversation
as I was in an alcove on the edge
of the ward.

What did I do all day?

I see myself as I was then
staring at the square of sky
in the window
straining to catch what nurses
and patients were saying
over there;
thinking ahead to the next meal;
wondering what kind of life
I will live
when I leave here.
Panicking that I will never work again
never be able to earn money
for the family.

That's a hole I disappear into
and I notice that I'm twiddling my toes
over and over and over again.

Here I know no one
and no one I know
can come and see me.

Here we get on with each other
only because we have bits wrong with us:
the guy with the stroke can't speak
but I point to his pot of Marmite
and give him a thumbs up.
He gives me a thumbs up back.

A man next to me
who I can't see
because I can't lift myself,
sings Caribbean songs
and listens to his wife talk to him
on the phone.

Another man over there
does the same:
I can hear his Irish wife on
his speakerphone
sounding like a beautiful James Joyce monologue
calling out:
'Is that a "yes", Jimmy? Is that a "yes"?'

In the morning I wave to him.
He can't speak but he does a smiley nod.

Another one struggles with his insides.
I hear the doctor
talking him through what isn't working.
It sounds like it's everything.

One guy
says he had gangrene
and they took his toes off.
He tells me that he used to lay tar,
he was a road-builder for thirty years,
but he gave it all up,
sold his house,
got rid of everything he had
and went on the road in France and Spain
with just one tiny one-man tent.
He keeps saying he's going to nip out
to the garden to have a fag.

I dwell on all these stories,
but try not to talk about me
in case I sound too un-ordinary.
I try not to be me.

One lets slip, just a day or two before he leaves,
that his father was a Jewish refugee
who fled from Hitler.
We swap stories of the trauma
our relatives went through.
We talk about Prague.
We both visited the Jewish cemetery.
Why didn't the Nazis destroy it? I ask.
As a memory of an extinct race, he says.
For a moment
it feels like I'm me, he's him,
but then he went.
The nurses stripped the bed
and laid stiff white sheets down.
I promise him I'll send him my book
about what happened to my father's uncles.
I make sure I've got his address.

They've been worried
about my low blood pressure
but they've brought me the Daily Mail
so it'll be fine in just a moment.

I watch the man opposite get up
grab a zimmer frame,
and walk slowly out of the ward,
holding it.
It seems so far from anything that
I can do.
Two people come to my bed
and say that they are going to get
me walking.
I am saddened by the feeling
that they are saying that to cheer me up
not because it's going to happen.

They tell me to swing my legs
out of the side of the bed.
They put a frame in front of me.
They tell me to push on the bed
behind me.
They help me grab the frame.
'One, two, three – let's go!' says the man.
I feel broken
I'm gasping for air.

They help me into a wheelchair.
That feels better:

I am pleasingly mobile,
I wheel to the window
and see the cars,
there's a man standing in his doorway,
a woman on a balcony,
watering her flowers.

Maybe I'm a wheelchair person from now on.
I practise taking corners,
pulling on one side and pushing on another.
I could be quite good at this.
I wheel down the corridor.
Nurses smile.
Yes, maybe I'm a wheelchair person.

I tell Emma on the phone that I've wheeled myself
down a corridor.
She says that when I come home
I'll be walking.
I think to myself (but don't say) that it won't
be like that.

The physios explain that
to get back into bed
I have to go from the wheelchair

to the zimmer to the edge of the bed.
They write this up on a chart above
the head of the bed.

We sit in the garden outside the hospital.
Emma has come with the children.
I'm in a wheelchair.
We wear masks and sun glasses.
We talk of cancelled holidays,
closed shops, lockdown,
What is this lockdown going on, I ask?
At least the weather was good,
they say.
But you wouldn't have noticed that,
they say.
What's the food like?
they say.
I like it,
I say,
especially the soups,
I think they liquidize the leftovers
from the day before.
Do you know something,
I say,
I can remember sometime
back at the other hospital
I couldn't feed myself,
my hands were shaking and
my arms were weak.

I know,
Emma says.
I think that means I've told her that
fifteen times before.

The physios say that they are taking me to the gym.
Again I work myself from the wheelchair
to the zimmer
and onto a padded bench.
They want me to stand up from the bench,
pushing with my hands behind me.
When I do, I am gasping again.
I hear my breath roaring in my right ear.
They tell me how to breathe:
in through the nose – deep and slow
out through the mouth – pursed lips.
They tell me that I have very low blood pressure
and my body doesn't want to stand up or walk.
Pedal your feet, they say, pedal.
I think of my heart wanting to take it easy:
every time it comes to the turn of the left ventricle
to pump blood round my body,
it thinks, why bother? Let's go back to bed
and lie down under the duvet.

But the physios want me to use the zimmer
to take a step.
I grip the zimmer
and try to lift my leg.
It feels as if I am asking a blank space

to work.
My foot shuffles a few inches.
The physios are pleased.
It feels as if they have expectations
way beyond what I'll ever do.
I wheel back to the bedside
lever on to the zimmer
and back into bed
and under the duvet.

Another day
the physios take me to some parallel bars.
I am allowed to grip them as I swing a leg,
or as I try to move forward
or sideways
or stand at one end
while we throw a ball to each other.
I feel a space in my middle
that hasn't worked for months.
I can walk a few steps with the zimmer.
I remember the man on our block
at home who must have had a stroke
who walks from his house to the shops
using a zimmer.
Maybe that's me from now on.
I remember that in the years I've seen him,
that's what he does. That's him.
He hasn't stopped using a zimmer.
That's where he's at.
Yes, maybe that's me.
Try not to shuffle, they say.
See if you can lift your feet up.
Look ahead.

1.

The bed sings:

'Why have you left me?

Come back.

I'm here for you.

Why do you waste your time

trying to move about

out there

when you could be lying soft

and still with me?

Come back

Come back

I will cover you with the gentle weight

of the furry blanket your wife sent me.

My pillow will stroke your cheek

Don't stand there alongside me,

weak and shaking.

I will hold you and support you

all day

all night long

Listen to me now:

remember me wherever you are.

In your moments of fear,

as you wonder if you can go on

with your crazy idea of wanting

to walk
you'll know I'm here
ready for you
for when you give up
give up
give up
give up'

2.
'No
I am learning to de-bed.
You have been good and kind to me
but I can't stay with you.
I will turn to mush
bits of me will stop
I will fade
I will slip into your folds
and never wake up again.
I am de-bedding myself.'

In the gym
I walk five steps
and grab the bar.
The physio says that's really good.
I'm proud.

She says that she knows
children who like my books.
I'm proud again
but then I'm sad.
I'm sure I won't be well enough
to stand in front of 500 children
ever again
telling them my poems and stories
hearing them laugh.
I say that to her.

She says that I can't say that.
Maybe you will do those things again, she says.

The Occupational Therapists taught me
how to own my frailty.
I have to choose:
do the work
or give up.

I put the therapists in my head every day.

The way I wrote that made it sound easy.

I meant to say:
it takes brain work
to stop saying, 'Help me'.

I do the work.

Emma comes to the gym
to watch me walk.
I'm getting anxious.
I want her to see that yesterday
I walked very nearly the whole length
of the gym, without stopping.
She sits on a bit of apparatus
and watches.
I hear myself panting again.
My legs go weak.
I'm not going to make it to the wall.
I sway and stop.
I was better yesterday, I say to her.
I hear that I'm pleading.
I glimpse myself years ahead
walking ten strides, gasping and stopping.
I'm not going to get better, am I?

Another day
they say that I'm not going to use the zimmer
anymore
and they give me an NHS stick:
aluminium, adjustable for height,
hard plastic handle.
I think that this is crazy.
I won't be able to support myself with just a stick.
The physios explain
that the way to move is
stick in the right hand
stick forward
left leg forward
right leg forward.
I can feel that they are holding me
Doreen the nurse is holding me
from behind.
I am doing that gasping thing again.
I am sure this is a pointless mission.
I was OK with the wheelchair
I was OK with the zimmer.
I don't need to do this stick thing.
They insist.

Stick. Left. Right.
Stick. Left. Right.
The stick shakes.
Keep your head up, they say.

This is dangerous.

I write a tweet
that I have a new friend,
Sticky McStickstick
and he is helping me walk.
It seems as if people are glad
that I'm not dead
and they are laughing about
Sticky McStickstick.
I take a photo of 'him'
lying in my bed,
handle on the pillow,
the shaft under the duvet.

Today, they say
we are going to try the stairs.
At the stairs
they tell me to grab the bannister
and haul myself up
first using one foot
and then the other.
My right leg won't do the work.
It refuses.
Don't worry this time, they say,
it'll come. Just use your left.
How many stairs have you got at home?
they say.
I try to imagine home
and the stairs.
It's hard.
I can't count them in my mind.
We want you to be able to climb stairs
before you go home, they say.
I think, why? I could live on one level.
I think of Chris's grandmother
living in the front room of their house.
But then I remember she was 90.
I'm 74.
Maybe I've become a kind of 90.

Someone said to me,
We're all the same age
but at different times.

I do the maths.
He's right.

I try to walk to the loo
without using Sticky McStickstick.
I stagger.
I think of:
M People, Heather Small:
I sing to myself
'Search for the hero inside yourself.'
When I get there
I sit on the loo
wondering how many people
have sung,
'Search for the hero inside yourself',
to get themselves to the loo.

The nurse tells Peter in the bed opposite,
that his urine is dark.
'The times are dark,' he says.

I know death.
I watched my mother die.
She sat up in bed, coughed,
a nurse jumped forward,
caught something that came out of her mouth
and she fell back against the pillows.

I went into my son's room
early one morning
to tell him that I was off out
but he was still and cold
and didn't hear me.
I rang 999
and they asked me to pull him
from the bed
and lie him on his side
and his arm stuck up in the air
away from his body
not moving
and when he landed on the floor
something came out of his mouth
on to the carpet.
They asked me to feel for his pulse.
There wasn't any.
I told them this

and they told me he was dead.
Later, they put him in a bag
I heard the zip
and they slid the bag down the stairs.

I realise that I've learned how to walk
three times:
the first,
I guess, was when I was about one
living in a flat over a shop
with a back yard.

I stayed walking every day
until I was 17:
I got knocked down by a car
spent 8 weeks in hospital in
a kind of hammock.
They told me to get up and walk.
I couldn't
so they sent me to a rehab centre
and taught me how to walk
in the middle of a field not far
from Watford.

And then after this Covid stuff.

Three times.
Seems a bit excessive.

A man comes on Saturday
and tells me he is the weekend physio.
He asks me to walk down the hospital corridor
using the stick.
I walk from the ward to the toilet and back
Stick, left, right.
I am pleased.
Maybe I could get to do more.
He says that I must be careful
that I don't become 'stick-reliant'.
I'm thinking how it's the stick
that's making it possible for me to walk.
Reliant is what I am.

In the gym
the weekday physios
are getting me to put the stick aside.
I am walking between the parallel bars,
I am allowed to touch them
but should try not to.
I manage that.
We are kicking a ball between us.
I imagine doing that at home
with my son the footballer.
That is so far away.
So far.

Your hands speak.
Touch is a language.
Each palm
each fingertip
is a line from your stories.

I get what they each say:
this hand is in a hurry,
this hand hesitates,
these hands are worried:
they catch me as I slope sideways.
This hand knows a lot:
it hunts for the lumps where previous jabs
filled me with blood thinner.
This hand hunts for bedsores:
it spreads Vaseline
and kindness.

In the middle of the night
I'm woken by nurses calling out,
switching on lights and pulling curtains.
I'm not sure if they are anxious or angry.
I listen in.
It seems as if someone has fallen
out of bed.
Are they blaming him?
Possibly. One of them calls out:
he was trying to walk!
I think none of us in here can walk,
we know that,
so perhaps he tried in his sleep.
I picture him behind the curtain
rolling sideways on to the floor.
I touch the metal rail along the side
of my bed.
It's like a fence, keeping me in.
I couldn't roll over that.
I guess that he must have moved his rail
to the dropped-down position.
The nurses are checking to see
if he's broken something.
I can't hear if he's saying anything to them.

Coming up to three months
I've been away.
Are you learning to live without me?
You must be making your morning coffee
and taking it upstairs yourself.
Is it good not to hear that noise I make
when I crunch that weird breakfast I concoct,
oats, 'Grape Nuts', raisins, raspberries?
Is it OK watching movies on TV
on your own?
Probably.
Is that paperwork I left behind
getting you down?
The accounts?
Maybe you don't hate
doing them as much as I do.
Are you getting sick of having
to tell people over and over again
how I am?
Is the bed bigger?

I carry the stick in my hand
and walk down the corridor without it.
I do it once.
I do it twice.
The physios say that before I'm discharged
they are going to come home with me
to see how I can get from room to room
how I can get upstairs
how I can get out and back into the house.

After 3 months I come home for a couple of hours
and the physios take me round the house,
showing me where to hold on to a rail
or use the wall,
and incredibly I see that
we do have a downstairs loo.
I had forgotten and had imagined that
every time I would need to go
when I was downstairs I would have to
haul myself up the stairs, panting and gasping.

The family watch me.
I wonder how it feels for them
to see me like this.
I am sorry this is me.

The physios say that they will send frames
to put next to the toilets so that I can pull myself up
and a bench to put across the bath so that I can
wash myself all over.

I walk into the living room.
I realise that they have taught me how to walk.
The gap between hospital and home
has closed.

VI.
GOING HOME

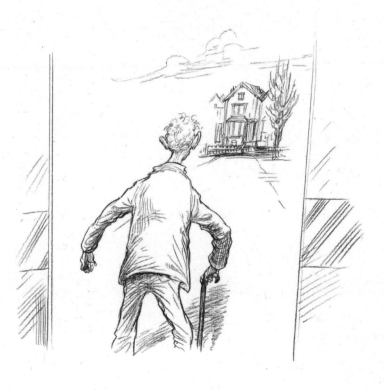

I am not sure I am me.
I can't see as I used to see.
I can't hear as I used to hear.
My legs feel like cardboard tubes,
filled with porridge.

I'm a traveller who reached
the Land of the Dead.
I broke the rule that said I had to stay.
I crossed back over the water,
I dodged the guard dog,
I came out.
I've returned.

I wander about.

I left some things down there.
It took bits of me as prisoner:
an ear and an eye.

They're waiting for me to come back.
The ear is listening.
The eye is the lookout.

My mouth has something in it
on the edge of my tooth at the back
next to my tongue.
I'm not doing what I have done
for the last 40 years – visit schools,
tell stories to hundreds of children
going into radio studios to interview
people about language
teaching students at universities.
I'm not that person.
I am someone sitting at home
wondering about the eye that can't see
the ear that can't hear
the tracheostomy wound that won't heal
the thing in my mouth.
I am someone trying to get stronger
by walking round and round the garden
or by lifting weights tied to my ankles.
I can hear myself trying to talk
as I used to
using the same words
putting my face into the same shapes
but it feels as if I am attaching myself
to things that don't belong to me anymore.
I'm not sure that I am me.

After I come home
I hear Emma saying
I was in intensive care for 47 days.
I think that when she told me that before
that I was in a ward where the care was intensive.
Just that.
Only after several times of her telling me this
do I get that much of the time
I was in an induced coma on a ventilator
with tubes coming in and out of me.
I realise that April and most of May have gone.
None of it is a memory.
There is nothing in my mind
from this time.
April and May.
She tells me that the nurses and doctors
sang me 'Happy Birthday' on May 7.
I think of her waiting at home
not knowing if I would live.
Not knowing whether even if I did live
whether I would come out of this a wreck.
I feel my face crumple
and I weep at the thought of her
holding firm.
All those days and nights.
And the children too.

Two physios come over.

They ask me to walk across the room.

They say that's very good.

They ask me to push my legs against their hands.

They say that's very good.

One of them asks me what are

my longterm objectives.

I stop and think.

What are my longterm objectives?

Do I have longterm objectives?

Should I have longterm objectives?

I would like to write a book

about a French dog called Gaston le Dog.

I don't say that.

I say that I would like to be able to

walk to the Jewish deli on the corner

and wheel the shopping back

in our trolley.

The physio smiles.

She writes it down in her book.

I'm trying to say that going shopping

and bringing it back

seems huge,

much bigger than anything I can do now.

It feels like a longterm objective.

Anything else? she says.
Live for a bit more? I think,
and I've never bothered to pickle cucumbers,
I just buy them,
but my mother made lovely pickled cucumbers,
I would like to try that one day.

You're doing very well, they say.

I've got a hole in my neck.
Emma explains that they put me to sleep
and made a hole in my neck
and put a tube in.
I remember dreaming of a white plastic chunk
in my throat
like a piece of penne pasta.
At home
I'm realising that
there were several times
when I could have died.
If Emma hadn't called the GP neighbour
if she hadn't tested me
I would have just faded away
a few hours later
all systems failing.
If the doctors hadn't put me on their machines:
ventilator and tracheostomy
I might have died for lack of oxygen,
if the nurses hadn't suctioned the secretions
out of my lungs
I might have drowned in my own phlegm,
if they hadn't played the music
that Emma had chosen
I might have stayed in a coma.

All those FaceTime phone calls
when she told me not to worry,
don't worry about a thing
how I was going to be OK
and she was telling people that I was
getting better
and I realised she was holding me,
propping me up with words.
All that care and belief and love
keeping me in the world.
I look at Emma
and try to tell her
but I'm often too upset to be able to say it
and just put my hand over my eyes
and feel the tears.

I've come out of this thing
lopsided:
my left eye is a blur
my left ear can't hear.
When I walk,
I feel as if my right side leads,
pulling the left side along.
I am not convinced that
my left foot is going where it should
so I look down
but then quickly feel myself tilt
leftwards.
My arm comes out to keep me from falling.
That works.

At the eye clinic
there are pieces of apparatus,
like little scaffolds sitting on a table:
silver and black.
Where I put my chin on the scaffold
there is a white plastic chin rest
and a white plastic bar
for me to lean my forehead against.
The apparatus clicks and clacks
as the doctor winches it upwards,
downwards, sideways,
I look into a lens
where lights like stained glass windows
in a darkened church appear:
red, yellow, blue.
A cross appears and disappears.
The doctor's face is a few inches away
on the other side of the apparatus.
He tells me to look at his ear.
I imagine days, weeks, months and years
of him asking people to look at his ear.
The lights shift, come into focus
and out again.
A red light comes close.
There's a blue cross

and a thin red line that moves gently
down the screen.
Later he shows me screen shots
of the inside of my eye:
of spheres, planets, distant stars
a streak of a comet caught mid-flight.
He points at a black hole.

I sit in a blue cubicle,
the doctor fits earphones on my head.
When I hear a beep I'm to press a button,
hold it down till it stops.
I shut my eyes.
I hear hissing.
I see the diagram of the ear in my mind
ear-drum, the hammer-anvil-stirrup bones,
the semi-circular canals, cochlea,
the auditory nerve.

Which bit of this beautiful organ is broken?
I hear a beep stop,
but I didn't hear it begin.
That means I missed pressing the button.
I try to tune in to the beep note.
That was a loud one.
I get the beginning and end of the next one.
I have a hope that after the test
the doctor will wiggle a poky thing around
in my ear, pull out a plug
and sound will stream in.
There goes another beep.
Keep my eyes shut.
All I have in my life at this moment

are the beeps.
I start to see them:
soft blue peas that pulsate.

The door opens.
He shows me graphs.
Good ear, bad ear.
The maths of my lopsidedness.
Maybe in a few months' time
I will find out what can be done –
if anything.
He rummages in his desk
and opens a white plastic box.
He digs out a curved grey tube
about the size of a small slug.
It's a hearing aid.
What? Now? Already?
He fits it into and over my ear,
connects it to an electronic device
round my neck
and it sounds as if
someone is shouting through a telephone
into the ear that's heard nothing
for months.
He talks of balancing the two ears.

He tweaks something from where he's sitting.
He shows me how to tweak the aid,
myself
using a tiny switch.
He gives me little trays of batteries.
They look like the pills
that I pop out of other little trays every morning.
These are silver.
He points at his screen and says that
the computer will tell him
when I am using the aid.
Maybe my aid talks to a satellite
which bounces back messages to him?

I want to say how grateful I am
but he's telling me that his daughter
loves my books.
I'm grateful that he's telling me that too.
As I walk away down the corridor
past the blue chairs
I feel less lopsided.
Emma says that we are dealing with
each thing bit by bit: eye, ear, trachy wound.
I mustn't think that everything will get done
straight away.

She is talking to me on the aid side.
A bit telephonish, I say
and then feel ungrateful for saying so.

Today I feel stupid.
I feel that I must have been stupid
to have caught Covid-19.
Streams of people I know come to mind
none of whom caught it.
I must have done something stupid.
There must have been some bit of knowledge
something I did unthinkingly
to be the only one.

And I feel this stupidity
has ended by my visiting it on Emma.
She gets the anticoagulant syringe ready
points the needle at the belt of fat round
my mid-riff
and sticks it in.
She pushes the syringe home
counts to ten
and pulls it out.
Why should she be doing this?
And the rest: the lifts to Outpatients,
the trips to the pharmacy, the phone calls
with doctors we can't see,

the shopping that I don't trust my legs to do
yet.
I've visited it on her
because I am stupid.

Sometimes I reverse the moments,
blurring the order of things.
Events come over the horizon
unattached to days or dates.
For a while it matters:
I try to get it straight:
did the moment when the inflow tube
into my mask fell off
come before I had to wear mittens
or after?

Keeping an order used to be important.
I used to say to my brother,
That holiday in Wales –
was it before we went to Northumberland
or after?

I'm beginning to think I don't need to know.
After all, if I did know
and I could line everything up,
chronologically,
chronologically,
how would it make anything easier?

You said that the last night I lay in the bed
struggling to breathe, you thought
the shadow of death crossed my face.
I remember the line about
walking
through the valley of the shadow of death,
or how the angel of death passes over some
and kills others.
I'm confused between thankful
and sorry,
thankful to be here now,
sorry for those who didn't make it,
sorry for you
as I imagine what it felt like
to look on that shadow.

There are 48 days of life
which are gone.
They are a nothingness.
Beyond recall.
A space I can't re-visit.
A time I can't daydream.
I take the pictures I have
of TV emergency shows:
grey and bruised people
with tubes up their noses
in their throats
drips on stands by their beds
monitors peaking, troughing
and bleeping,
and put myself in the beds.

It's make-believe.
I don't know that I lived that.
It was a pre-death.
A rehearsal for the real thing,
which I didn't take part in.
I was there, you tell me.
But not there.

The house is old.
There's a crack on the wall.
We'd better find someone to look at that.
Difficult to know if it's serious
– 'structural' –
or just a hairline job in the plaster.
Difficult to say just from looking at it.
There are places where the paint
has chipped.
Can they be touched up
or does that whole area need painting?
Some of the nails in the boards
are rising.
Doesn't matter much
but there could be a knock-on effect
if one of us is in bare feet.
Funny how damage in one place
can lead to damage somewhere else.
One of the taps is leaking.
There are one or two tiles on the roof
that have slipped.
The house is old.

I shower.
Hair first.
I love the hot water embrace.

I draw my hand down over my face
and feel hairs in my mouth.
I let the water help wash them away,
down to the shower tray.
It's a coil.

I do it again.
Down off my hair
over my face.
The water washes another coil
onto the tray.
I lay the coils out on the rim
of the tray.

After I've washed the rest of me,
and dried off,
I go and get a couple of pages
of loo roll,
come back to the shower-tray rim,
gather up the coils with the pages
take the package to the loo

and flush it away.
I come back to the bathroom mirror.
I see skin between the hairs
on the top of my head.
I think it's best not to try
a comb-over.

1.

Every morning:
I rub my right hand in the thyme plant
that Emma has put on the balcony
and then bring my fingers to my nose
and breathe in.

2.

Sunday treat:
added a spoonful of honey
to my lemon tea.

3.

That feeling:
when the postman says,
'Good to see you up and about.'

vii.
RECOVERY

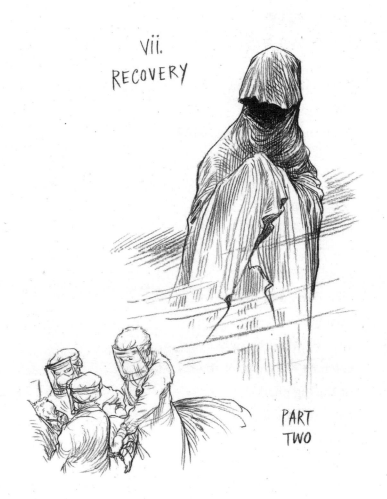

PART
TWO

I am not who I was.
I am who I was.
This is not me.
This is me.

I am now the person
who had Covid:
the thing that came in March

I am now the person
who disappeared
in April and May

I am now the person
who peers into the mirror
hoping his left eye
will see what the right eye sees,
catching a glimpse of the blackness
of the big pupil
looking back at me in hope.

I am now the person
who hears the telephonic trebly sound
through the hearing aid
in his left ear,

that makes the sound of a kettle boiling
into scream.

I am now the person
who is alert to every twinge
or mark anywhere on me.
I am getting to know this person.
This is not me
This is me

I meet the consultant who was in charge
of intensive care.
He tells me it was carnage.
People were dying all round me.
I wasn't dying
but they didn't know if I would wake up.

He tells me about Covid-19
and his words create a picture of a spike
from the virus attaching itself to a protein
in us:
he demonstrates it with his finger hitting
his fist.

The virus seems so clever:
it takes advantage of how our bodies react,
going through our lungs
and wrecking organs all over us.
It's hard not to think of it as having
intent, that it is doing things
because it wants to.
Tiny viruses with enormous brains.
I've looked at pictures of it:
blue and spiky.
In my mind it's become a wicked hedgehog.

I tell myself this is neither scientific
nor helpful.

The consultant tells me that Emma
did it.
They had tried to wake me up.
She had told them what music I liked.
She sent them in pictures of the family.
I opened my eyes
but they weren't sure I could see
and I waved my arms about
as if I was agitated about something
but I wasn't awake.

They didn't know if I would wake up.

He told me they arranged a meeting.
I was wheeled out.
Emma came in.
She talked to me.
She squeezed my hand.
She played me messages from the children.

Emma has told me this, I think.
But then he says, we wheeled you into the lift

and you were transformed,
you were awake and you understood
what was going on.
That was the breakthrough moment.

I am washed over with knowing
that the things she said and did
reached into a mind that was frozen
and untrapped it.
She freed me.

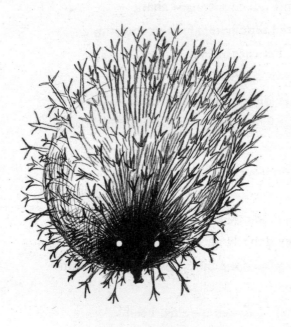

WICKED HEDGEHOG

I think about two cliches today:

ignorance is bliss
a little learning is a dangerous thing

I remember in hospital
nurses and doctors telling me things
about me.
I had no idea whether this meant
that I'd be dead the next day.
I have the feeling now that
at the time
I didn't care.
Maybe it was the meds they were giving me.
I had a built-in shrug.
You've got microclots in the brain, they said.
So what?
If they're micro, I thought,
I'm not going to get agitated about them.
I can't see them.
They don't hurt.
I didn't look up 'microclots on the brain'.

Things I thought were crucial,
like my foggy eye,

the doctors didn't seem bothered about.
But everything's lopsided, I say,
I can't see properly.
I can't read.
This is the first time we've heard of foggy eye
as a result of Covid, said one young doctor.
I thought: I don't really care
if it is the first time,
but I would love it if we could do something
about it.

Now I'm home,
the moment something new happens:
my knee joint hurts, spots come up on my good eye,
my right nipple is sore –
I open up the computer and fill my mind
with possible causes, possible outcomes,
possible dangers.
I trawl through side effects of each drug
in the symphony of drugs by the bedside.

Occasional side effect of finasteride:
sore nipple.

Now I know.

That's that one solved.

But is it?

Is there another cause for sore nipple?

I google 'sore nipple'.

It's midnight.

I should go to sleep.

I wonder about another timeline:
not my own.
When did the World Health Organization
tell us a pandemic was on the way?
When did they tell us about the need for
masks and social distancing;
test and trace?

I go to the website and find February.
For the first time I feel angry.
I want to know why our government
didn't do what the WHO said
every country should do?
It seems as if they thought they knew better.
I read of more sinister ideas:
that they would allow some of us to die
in the wave of virus flowing over the population
because everyone else would get 'immunity'.
Those of us who died
would be the price worth paying.
And anyway, the most likely to die
are old and sick, so they (we?)
matter less than the young and fit?

My mind goes back to when I got ill.
If the government had done what the WHO

suggested, I wonder,

perhaps these things wouldn't have happened

to me,

nor to the thousands of others like me,

nor to the thousands who've died.

Today I walk to the dentist.

The hygienist scrapes and polishes

my teeth

from behind a mask and a screen.

From the dentist I walk on to the supermarket.

I buy some porridge oats for us

and croissants for Emma and the children.

I get confused at the checkout.

The assistant helps me.

I walk home.

'I've bought you a present,'

I say to Emma.

Tomorrow I am going further:

to Martyn's

the shop that sells the best dried fruit

the best pickles, the best fruit cakes,

the best oaty biscuits in the world.

I will buy giant yellow sultanas for me

and chocolate gingers for Emma.

The supplies are in:
pills, syringes, eye drops, ointments,
gels, mouth washes.
I have weights and a cycling machine for exercises
and a band that I stretch for 'resistance'.
We could buy a blood pressure machine
and an oximeter to measure me
as I sit, stand, or climb the stairs.
Maybe there are self-help x-ray machines
and MRI scanners
that we could set up in the living room.
I remember saying to the nurse
that my drip wasn't working.
It's not dripping, I said.
We could have one of those too,
the metal stand beside me at the kitchen table
as we eat our Friday night take-aways.

At the scan
they ask me if I have any metal implants.
I say no.
When I get home,
I remember when I was a kid
I swallowed a little metal leg off
my father's portable alarm clock.
What if it was still there?
It could have wrecked the scan.

The boxes of pills
pile up beside the bed
like kiddies' blocks.
This one, three times a day,
this one once a day,
this one, two times a day.
Each box labelled with
jazzy names:
Apixaban, Finasteride,
Nitrofurantoin, Levothyroxine.
I read the accompanying leaflet:
possible side effects –
always diarrhoea.
Why isn't a possible side effect
uncontrollable laughter,
or a desire to play bass guitar?

There are eye drops:
Dexamethasone
Dorzolamide
Bimatoprost/Timolol.
Three times a day
for two weeks,
two times a day for one week.
Or is it the other way round?

Emma knows.
'Put your head back.'
Squirt.
They feel like shampoo in the eye.
It stays cloudy.
The consultant will tell me about
glaucoma
and say, 30 is not good.

I learn new names
anterior chamber
anticoagulant
ureter
oedema
medial ligament.

I remember that I tried to be a doctor.
I learned about the oxygen dissociation curve
and Krebs cycle.
I even saw Krebs once.
A little old man, bent over,
leading students through the lab.
Holocaust survivor.

But I couldn't do it.
I found that I didn't love it enough.

But here I am
rolling anticoagulant apixaban
round my mouth
like I know what I'm talking about.
Stop it, Michael.
You're not a doctor.
You're a patient.

One med I take four times a day.
Three meds I take two times a day.
Three meds I take once a day.
One of the three meds I take once a day
in two doses.

We used to say that we didn't like the noise
of the air condition vent of La Luna cafe,
out the back of our house.
It's on today, as usual:
a steady breathy hum.

We used to say that we would call the council
to see if it was over the limit of permissible noise.

Maybe we'll do that.

I notice that the noise blocks out
the hiss in my deaf ear.

For a moment
I'm not so sure that we should call the council
just yet.

We tell people that I am home.
It's in the papers,
I am on the radio and TV.
Michael is home.

People are delighted and send kind messages.
Some of them say
how glad they are that I have recovered.
Some say they are glad that
I am back to my old self.

I'm glad they are glad.
I feel lucky that people care.

I look at the word 'recovered'.
I want to change it to 'recovering'.
I'm not sure that I will be 'recovered'.
As for that old self,
he's that guy I knew six months ago

Our daughter tells me that
when you talked to me
on FaceTime,
when I was in Intensive Care,
my eyes were open,
but I just stared,
not speaking,
not responding to what you said.

I am getting it that
there is a place
between life and death.

I was there for weeks.

The more I find out
about the state I was in
before I got to A and E;
the more I find out
about the state I was in
in intensive care,
I get it that there were several times
I could have just faded away.
Perhaps I shouldn't have tried so hard
to find out.

Years ago, I sat by my children's beds
waiting for a fever to go.
I'm a parent.
It's what we do.

The nurses have given me a 'Patient Diary'.
Reading it, I get to realise that
as I lay there unconscious
a nurse sat by my bed
all night,
night after night
talking to me,
telling me things,
cleaning me;
trying to wake me up out of the coma,
and then when the long night
was over
they sat and wrote me a letter
to put in this 'Patient Diary'.

I try to fathom
this devotion.
They aren't my parents.

I read how bus drivers died
because the government ordered the lockdown
one week too late.
Bus drivers: sitting in their cabs being breathed on
by hundreds of people every day
and dying.
And it could have been avoided.
They could be with their partners, children,
friends, workmates.
I feel hot and angry.
It is unjust.
But let's not talk about death.
Let's talk about life.
Hundreds of people helped me have that.
I bathe myself in the stories
that Emma tells me of what she said
and did while I was so nearly gone.
Do you know she sent in a duvet
so that I didn't have to try to keep warm
with the thin blue sheets
that the hospital calls 'blankets'?
Have I told you that before?
I repeat myself a lot.
But some people didn't know me.
Many people.

Many of them spoke to me with voices
tuned in countries far from here.
For a moment it feels as if they travelled
thousands of miles from home
just to save my life:
Brazil, Nigeria, Grenada, Uganda, Philippines,

I read their diary-letters to me
that they wrote
in a little black book when I was in the coma.
Why did these strangers try so hard
to keep me alive?
It's a kindness I can hardly grasp.
The words tell me
that they wanted me to survive.

I may never meet them again.
Let's talk about life.

The Radio Four Today Programme
saw a tweet I wrote about
how people seemed to be talking
as if it wouldn't matter too much
if old people died of Covid-19
or at least
not as much as young people.
I had written that this felt wrong
as if now that I was over 70
I was dispensable.

They asked me to come in
and talk about this on the Today Programme.

And I did.

I said that I wanted to live.

This was March 10.

This means that as I was saying this
I was already infected with Covid-19.

I think of my father's last years
how he shrank down to a list of ailments:
which bit of him hurt
which bit of him had been removed
which bit of him that was left.

He tried to talk of other things:
he recommended a book for me to read
a week before he died.
We did sometimes talk football.
He did ask after the children
but he soon returned to what really
interested him:
the bit of him that hurt
the bit of him that had been removed
the bit of him that was left.

Before he got really ill
we used to talk about the book
he was writing.
When I was 13 he read us 'Great Expectations'
with all the voices,
later: 'Catch-22' and 'Catcher in the Rye'
and even later, his own short stories.
He raved about old foreign authors:

Isaac Babel, Alexander Herzen,
Anton Makarenko
like they were his friends.
His eye was like a headlight
pouring over upcoming landscapes.
He felt entitled to explore the world.

But then he shrank
and the landscape that he examined
and feared the most
was the bits of his body.

I tell myself that I see the danger.
Listen to me going on and on
about my eye, my ear,
the anticoagulants.
Oh today I'm feeling weak.
Oh today I'm feeling less weak.
Oh today it's my knee.
Oh today my toes are numb.
I hear myself shrink.

I see in a moment that surprises me today
that I don't know you, Connie, my mother
half as much as Harold,
your husband, my father.
You went when you were 56,
that's over 44 years ago.
There are clear scenes that
I repeat:
us laughing at a joke
about fermented banana
in a book
called 'Miskito Boy' that
you were reading to me in bed.
Your rare irritations with my
teenage long hair
when you would frown and turn
away from me with a move of
your head.

I have your articles and papers
and the book that you wrote with
Harold.
I see times when you two were
writing that, you didn't like what
he wanted to write, and you said so.
That couldn't have been easy.

In your last months, when you
hated what you looked like
because the doctors had taken
away half your jaw, we didn't talk,
did we? Women I hardly knew
came to the house,
went into your room and shut the door.
They came out hours later
and left.
I've wondered what you talked about
and now I don't remember the names
of the women who came.
I know you had hopes to do more,
you weren't finished –
far from it,
you wanted to carry on with
the people who studied with you
and learned new ways of doing things;
they write to me sometimes
to tell me how much their time
with you mattered.
You've lasted.

And now I remember
that thing you said to me,
where the Yiddish you spoke as a child

(and sometimes rejected)
broke through:
you were cross that a good idea
could, in the wrong hands, go bad
so you said,
'Michael, even the best ideas
some people will turn into dreck.'

Just before you died
you said, 'I've had a good innings,
haven't I?'
You who never played cricket,
didn't watch it on TV
didn't talk about it when
Harold and I got excited about
Jim Laker getting 19 wickets,
in one Test match,
you who must have had in the back
of your mind a hundred Yiddish phrases
about life and death,
turned to cricket for words
to say what it had all been for.

And I don't know why you did.

'dreck': shit

The air is full of vaccinations and cures.
We are offered pictures of labs,
pipettes, syringes,
and masked scientists
moving silently behind layers of glass
like fish.

There's news of people being vaccinated
in distant places,
told to us with suspicion and doubt.

We wait,
looking in on the aquariums.

I remember going to see the doctor
about a spot on my leg:

Me: I've got a spot on my leg.
Doctor: What do you think it is?
Me: Skin cancer?
Doctor: It's more serious than that.
Me: Really?
Doctor: It's old age.

There's a thin tube
that runs from the hearing aid
to the earpiece in my ear.
The audiologist gave me
a bit of plastic wire
and said that I should clean out
the tube with it.

Every now and then
my hearing aid
stops working
so I thread the bit of plastic wire
down the tube and it shunts
a bit of my earwax out.

It's very satisfying.

My dentist: You have teeth,
then fillings, then crowns,
then extractions,
then dentures.
Me: Then you die.
My dentist: Yes.

My son has discovered a new game:
coming up behind me
cupping his hands over my hearing aid
and moving them to and fro at speed
so that it gives out a tinny roar
to whatever rhythm he makes with his hands.

Walking against the wind today
was
phoooophhh
woooophhh
shwoooophhh
barooooophhh.

JF writes: hope you're making giant strides
I reply: The strides are pretty big.
Thanks.
I'm better walking down slopes than up them.
This causes problems for getting home
having been out.
Trouble with Muswell Hill where I live,
there's a hill.
I suppose the clue's in the name.
Everywhere round here is either up or down.
It's very bad geography behaviour.

If it's a road,
I got very nearly to the end.
But then people, many people
pulled me back.
They wouldn't let me go.
They worked harder than me:
incisions, tubes, drips,
pumps, ventilator.
They sat beside my bed
making sure that I didn't
head off to the end of the road again.

I just lay there sleeping
and absorbing.
And absorbing.

There's no destination, someone says to me,
there's only the journey.

Dear children,

I got ill.
We get ill.
You get ill.

I'm getting over it,
on the mend
people say.

I'm doing my best,
like you do your best.

I don't know how it will work out.
We never know for certain.
That's the one thing we do know
for certain:
that we never know for certain!

What we always have is now.
The moment before the next moment.
It's only the next moment
we're not sure about.

So whatever we've got to do
we have to do it now.

In the moment that we have for certain.

That's what I'm trying to do.
I can see you're doing things too.
You're doing them now.
That's good.
It's the only time you can do them.
But you know that.

Lots and lots of love
Dad.

Stop frowning, Michael.

Too much frowning.

Stop it.

Part of my medical report today
says that I was 'lyrical'.
Just as well.
All that English Literature I studied.
It would be really worrying
if they said I was 'unlyrical'.

In this time
this time of lockdowns,
social distancing,
and masks,
I don't meet doctors.
We do telephone appointments.

So there's no touching
no pulse taking
no blood pressures
or temperatures.

I get through and the doctor says
'How can I help you?'
I explain that something strange
is going on:
I get a feeling that starts behind my eyes
spreads through my body
like a hot flush
and ends with me wetting myself.

There's a pause.

'What medication are you on?'

I think, she should know what
medication I'm on.
There's a long list of stuff
for all the different bits of me
that they say need propping up,
reducing, or curing.
I start to reel them off.
'Ah yes,' she says, reading from a computer screen
'I've got them here.'
I ask her if she thinks any of that cocktail
of pills, ointments and drops
could be causing this?
She says no.
Could it be linked to any of the other things
going on – the numb toes, the eyes, the bits of extra
bone I seem to be growing?
She says no.

I'm on the phone.
She is on the phone.
This doesn't feel like an 'appointment'.
It feels like my father talking to me
on the phone
about the colour of his pee
as if I really did turn out to be the doctor
he always hoped I would become.

She makes a diagnosis:
I've got a urinary infection.
I always call it my 'waterworks'.
Urinary infection sounds more serious.
She prescribes a pill.
I remind her that I'm taking all the other pills
and drops and ointments
and hadn't we better check that this pill
doesn't clash with all the others?
She checks.
Oh dear.
It does clash.
She prescribes another.
'And come to the door of the surgery
pick up a bottle
and give us a sample.'
She means pee into the bottle
so that they can find out if she's right.
They'll send that off to a lab.
There'll be a number.
She'll put that into the computer.
'You have got a lot going on, haven't you?'
she says.
Yes, I say.
'That's what we're finding out with Covid,'

she says.
Yes, I say.
She wishes me well
and the phone conversation ends.

My legs have become maps
I can trace rivers in these veins,
though I follow them down to my feet
when my head knows
that no matter how slowly
and reluctantly they do it,
they flow up.

I remember the name of the place
they're going to:
the right auricle.
I remember how I remembered
what arteries do:
a is for artery
and a is for away from the heart
so even the joker in the pack,
the one artery that carries blood
without a cargo of oxygen,
flows 'away' from the heart,
marking out a route from the right ventricle
to the lungs,
all places that the internet
tells me could have been damaged.

Every time I get up out of a chair
the physiotherapist in me
left over from the Rehab hospital
says,
'Nose over toes'.

I'm having a blood test.
The nurse asks me to clench my fist,
she looks for the vein.
I watch the point of the needle hover over
the faint lines in the crease
of my arm.
In it goes.
I follow my blood moving down the tube.
In a moment
she will pull the needle out,
press a pad of cotton wool on the snick
in my skin,
then peel off some micropore tape
and stick it over the top.
It comes into my mind that I'm on blood-thinning
pills:
instructions full of grave words about
nose bleeds and bruises.
I think that
slicing tomatoes is life-threatening.
Now here's someone making a hole in me
and sucking out blood.
It's dark.
But will it stop?
Perhaps I will empty out through

the needle's perforation in the vein,
drop by drop
for days.
And days.
There, she says, all done.
Outside, I lift the cotton wool pad
to get a glimpse of the torrent gushing
out of my arm.
There's no mark.
Not even the usual blot.
Nothing.
I haven't bled to death.

Either Covid or intensive care
took away my big toe nails.
One's growing back.
The other one isn't.
This helps me work out
if big toe nails matter
or not.

Someone writes me a tweet about lockdown:

'I care, right now,
about the kids in the country
and how badly they are being affected
by this ridiculous imprisonment.
You should care about them too,
if you are half the man you used to be.'

I reply;
'I'm not half the man I used to be.
I'm busy trying not to be dead.'

Trace?

No one has ever asked me
where I was
or who I was with.

There are people
on the internet
trying to tell me that
I'm a hoax, or I've been hoaxed
or I'm part of a plot or
I've been plotted against.
It's all a trick to take away our freedoms
and make money from masks
or something.

I suppose there's a way of thinking that
clouds are a conspiracy
against the sun,
if you want.

They've announced
that schools will be reopening in September.

There must be evidence coming in
that the Coronavirus only travels
as far as the school gates,
gets sulky,
turns round
and hurries off.

The coma keeps secrets.
There is no place for the coma in
the geography of my memory.
I can't visit the coma.
I can't call for it.
If I try to find it,
if I plead for it to come,
it doesn't hear.
Or if it hears,
it refuses to come out of its cave
and tell me what happened.
It hangs back in the shadows
forbidding me from
having a conversation.
There isn't even a sign saying:
'This is not a memory'.

I realise that I've forgotten his name.
He is unbelievably famous.
He is in hundreds of films.
We talked about him yesterday.
We laughed about how
he's always running
he's always the good guy
he's always the one who figures out
what's wrong with the bad guys
I remember that clip of him
talking about Scientology
I remember him on the Graham Norton Show
leaning forward keenly.
I remember him in 'Magnolia'
and 'The Firm'.
We talked about him yesterday
how he figured out that the bad guys
were on some kind of tax fiddle,
wasn't that it?
Not him of course, but the character
he was playing
though there has come a point
that he's been in so many films like that
I'm beginning to think it's him
who's doing it.

Yesterday you said his name.

I said his name.

Today I can't remember it.

Islands of memory
Seas of forgetting
Islands of memory
Seas of forgetting
Islands of memory
Seas of forgetting

In about six weeks
I've lost most of the hair off the top of my head.
I've gone bald.
We look at the side effects of the meds:
none of them mention baldness.
One of them says that you may grow hair
in places where hair doesn't usually grow.
Like where?
On the palms of my hands?
But nothing about going bald.
Emma finds an article about hair falling out
as a response to shock and trauma.
I guess I had some of that.
It'll grow back, she says.
Unlikely, I think.

I watch some football on TV
to stop myself thinking about this stuff.
There's Pep Guardiola, manager of Man City:
not a hair on his head.

My teenage son feels that it's his right
to punch me,
if he gets a football score prediction
right and I get it wrong.
'I'm right, and you're wrong,' he says,
'what are you?'
'Wrong,' I say.
'What are you?' he says.
'Wrong,' I say.
Now the next thing coming up is the punch.
I put my hand up.
'You can't punch me,' I say.
'I'm on blood thinners.
If you punch me, you'll bruise me
and I will bleed to death very, very slowly
from the inside.'
It stops him from punching me.
'What are you?' he says.
'Wrong,' I say.

Clothing tip:
if you drop a blob of hummus by mistake
on your crocs,
make sure
that it doesn't land on one of the holes.

We are at a motorway service station
there are arrows on the floor
and lines for keeping a 'safe distance'
one for Costa
one for McDonald's
a sign for the toilets
about not going in if it's crowded
people are coming in
and going out
I pinch my mask over my nose
I hear voices in my hearing aid
voices that I don't hear with my good ear
I feel as if I shouldn't be standing
where I'm standing
which is in front of an arcade of slot machines
which make trilling noises.
You've gone over to a sandwich place
I think.
I'm holding an egg mayo sandwich
and a flapjack.
I am confused without knowing
what I'm confused about.

Before all this,
the body was reliable.
It told me stories of good walks,
swimming for an hour,
running round a field.

I knew its damage:
a corned-beef can
that sliced my thumb
a cricket ball that broke my nose,
a hole they call a hernia.

These things were stitched up
slotted back into place.

Now
the body is unreliable.
The stories it tells
are hard to believe.
There was something in me
that clotted blood,
stopped nerves working,
invaded my ear and eye
and veins.

I used to tell my students about
the 'unreliable narrator'
the one who tells the story
but can't be believed.
My body is an unreliable narrator.

I go online to read news of what the virus
is doing today.
How many lungs has it got into?
Millions.
This must make it one of the most successful
viruses ever.
It's won a virus race.
Though it can kill its host,
enough carriers are alive and coughing
chalking up yet more successes for Covid-19.
There I go again:
talking of a virus as if it knows what success is.
A scientist peers out of his video link
into the BBC Newsnight studio and says,
It's not even living. It's a virus,
it can't reproduce without a host.
A bit like grown-up children
who themselves have children
while still living with their parents.

The consultant says that
I'm going to have a Xen operation,
on my eye.
I hear it as a Zen operation.
I imagine standing in an operating theatre:
we meditate on the eyeball.
We chant:
cornea
cornea
anterior chamber
anterior chamber
optic nerve
optic nerve
retina
retina

The consultant explains that
it's x,e,n,
they're going to put
a tube in my eye.
This will drain my eyeball.

I think of the tube that Roald Dahl
helped invent
that they put in the back of his son's head

after his accident
to help it drain the fluid off his brain.

The consultant is worried about
the pressure in my eye.
When he says this,
I see my eye swelling up and bursting.

Someone posts a tweet saying
some of the Covid stories are
untrue, lurid and unnecessarily scare people.

I post back:
I made up my Covid story.
In reality I was hiding under the table.

The person replies:
Of course I wasn't saying
you made up your Covid infection
but you're 74.

'But you're 74'.

I think about 'but'.
What is 'but' about being 74?

Sweet sleep

I need you, I know.

Sweet sleep

I know I need you

when my face feels the pillow.

Sweet sleep

you wash away the wants and wishes

Sweet sleep

you are the place I need to go

Sweet sleep

Dream

We were at Land's End.
We climbed over a stone wall.
On the other side,
I noticed that we were at the top of a cliff:
sheer drop, hundreds of feet down.
I said that I wanted to go back
over the wall
but I noticed a big hole in the wall.
I squeezed into it so that I could get through
but got stuck.
I shouted to you: 'Push, Emma! Push!'
You did.
But I couldn't get through.
Then I noticed that there were people
walking around.
It was a space like a ruined church
made suitable for visitors
with surfaced walkways.
I called out to someone:
'Can you pull me through?'
He tried but he couldn't.
I felt so helpless
and I was worried about you

at the top of that cliff.
You were still pushing.
Then I called out to another person
in the ruined church.
He got hold of me
and pulled me through.

Did my ear scan at hospital just now.
They squeezed me into a confined space,
slid me into a tunnel
and smothered me in humming and drumming noises.
Quite familiar really:
almost identical to the London Underground.

No results from my scans yet,
but I've been summoned to have an echocardigan.
I mean echocardiogram.

An echocardiogram:
I lie on my side,
bare-chested,
sticky pads monitoring me.
I wonder if the echocardiographer
is from Barbados.
He commentates on my heart:
'Left ventricle 65%.
Well done.'
I feel proud.
As if I did it.
Then again, thinking about it,
I did.
It is my ventricle.

Now it speaks:
a watery gloop.
Or is that a ta-ta-gloop?
I listen to me.

We are a collection of tubes and pipes.

Some big.

Some tiny.

Sometimes the plumbing goes wrong

or a pipe gets blocked.

I've become wild and carefree
about what places I stop at
to put in my eye drops.
(Every two hours at the mo.)
No longer hide-in-the-bedroom, me.
I can stop in the street now.
Blop.
Done.

Waiting for the microwave to finish
used to be so boring,
but it's become the timer
for a quick glutes workout,
or holding the mini-squats position.
I've un-boringed the microwave.

Woman at the door asks me
if I want anything sharpening.
My wits, I say.

(I didn't.
My wits aren't sharp enough)

Off to the Ear Nose and Throat clinic.
It's an appointment with the three fates:
Ear, Nose and Throat.
An old plaque on the wall explains that
it was once the Royal Ear Hospital.
A hospital for the Royal Ear.

On floor Minus One,
they push a probe up my nose
and down my throat.
They show me the pics.
It looks like I've swallowed a squid.

The trick about going to sleep
is to make peace with
the landscape of my body.
Each of the irks and tweaks:
toes, knee, eye, tailbone, veins
must be smoothed away.
Stop fighting them.
Nothing must matter.
Where there are twinges
there can only be nothings.
All that's left is breath.
Feeling it drawn in through
the base of my back
feeling it flow out
between my teeth
feeling my stomach
flatten
over and over and over
till the landscape
is at peace
and asleep.

I climb the stairs.
Yes, I've climbed them every day
since I've been home
but now,
I'm climbing them for the first time
without touching the bannister.

I topple,
but just avoid the touch.
I wobble forwards,
but don't touch the stair.
My right leg caves leftwards
but I play the tightrope walker
and balance myself with my arms.

I get to the top
and walk towards the loo
panting.

I hear my breaths,
and think of how
even climbing stairs has come to matter
so much.

I must not expect you dear children
to be excited by this.

Not even to be mildly pleased.
Let's just go on.

Tightrope walker.
As if.

The wind is coming off the sea,
breakers punching the shore,
a man and a woman on chairs
watching the sea rolling towards them,
their children hiding behind their chairs.

The man and the woman are still.
The children crouch,
protected from the wind
behind their parents in their chairs.

I lie on a blanket
another one over me.
I seem to be below the wind.
I close my eyes.

I open them
the man and the woman and the children
are still there.

The sun breaks up on the waves.

It's been a good day.

I walk the beach
testing each step
for safe enough sand:
fear of toppling.
I make it to the cliff,
look up at its massiveness.
A child
leaps from one rock to the next,
hulks in the sand
ignoring her whoops of delight.
The sea gets on with
doing what it's always done.

A week later
the News tells of a cliff fall.
It was at that beach.

I pick out four bowls from the dishwasher
walk strongly
across the kitchen with my arms outstretched,
deep breathing,
feel my abs take the pressure.
I go back for the cups.
Carry them to the cupboard
arms outstretched
feel the muscles again.
I go back for a big bowl
bend the knees,
kneecaps over toes
this is good for vastus medialis,
surely.
I hold a saucepan behind me
raise and lower
raise and lower:
triceps? Must be.

A few days later
I tell the NHS physio
about my dishwasher workout.
She smiles – more to herself
than to me.
I guess she is thinking

doing exercises is great
but perhaps not all the time?
Life is not an exercise.

I wrote a poem 'No breathing in class!'
where I say that
we had a teacher who was so strict
we weren't allowed to breathe in class.
She used to say to us:
'NO BREATHING!'

Today I have what's known as a Xen op:
the surgeon is going to insert a tiny tube
into my eye to help it drain and get rid of glaucoma.
He has already told me his son likes my stuff
and has shown him a tweet
where I said that I was going to have an eye op today
where they were going to take my eyeball out,
stick it in the hospital washing machine
and then fix it back with superglue.
Here's what happens next:

I'm gowned up,
my eye fixed open,
all the overhead lights are on,
the nurses are gathered round,
it's the pause before the surgeon
is going in to the eyeball
and he says to me: 'No breathing.'

When I first heard
there was a band called Half Man Half Biscuit
I nearly wept at the joyous originality of it.
I've always tried to think up
new Half Man descriptions of me.
I've got it now:
Half Man Half Blood Clot.

At the eye clinic
the surgeon tells me
that the tube he put in my eye
is working very well.
The fluid has got somewhere
to go now, he says.

I have a drainpipe in my eye.

Eye clinic again:
second one in two days.

I have to look through a pin hole.
Oh the letters I see!
A lovely H.
And a W.
And a K.

Though it could be an R.

The voice therapist overseeing my recovery
from the tracheostomy
says I shouldn't clear my throat.

Instead: bend my head down
and swallow.

And I have to make foghorn noises
with my hand over my mouth.
To strengthen my voice,
I've got to make it difficult for myself
to make foghorn noises.

And no throat clearing.

Yesterday was a first:
I talked to my students on 'Zoom'.
It was about 'The Water Babies':
a world underwater
where children who run away
survive.

Yesterday I also thought how
the space in my head
where Eddie lives –
(now he's been gone for more than 20 years)
has become untended.

In a dream last night
I was in a swimming pool.
Eddie did an underwater handstand.
I heard him shouting from down there.
He came up
his face under a waterfall
of swimming pool water.
I asked him if he was ok.
He laughed.
The shouting underwater
was one of his tricks.
He always liked to see me
worried about whether he was ok.

Dizzy days.
Some days are dizzy.
Things swing around
inside my skull.
I sway.
I catch myself sloping sideways.
Is it down to those arches in my ear
they call the 'semi-circular canals'?
Today I think the virus got in there too.
It nosed about,
then set up camp.
The delicate balance system
doesn't know up from down.
It struggles to keep up with
my decisions to nod
or lie flat.
The canal flow has slowed.
The virus turned it to treacle,
I think.

Ear, Nose and Throat call me.
They say that microbleeds in my brain
damaged my auditory nerve.
I hear this through the phone
that I've put to my right ear.
The doctor asks me to take the hearing aid
off my left ear.
'Now put the phone to that ear,' she says.
I hear her call out: 'Ninety-nine'.
Then there's a faint rustle –
along with the sea-shell hiss
that keeps me company now.
I put the phone back to my right ear.
'I heard you say "ninety nine",' I say,
'and not much else.'
She talks to me about megahertz:
I still have a narrow band of them in my left ear.
The rest have gone.
The hearing aid does its best with the leftovers.
I'm guessing the microbleeding stopped.
The greyness in a corner of my brain
must have turned red.
And perhaps now it's brown.
Haemorrhage.
As hard to spell as diarrhoea.

What I didn't do just then:
walk back down the road
to white van man
(who was hooting me
because the cab that brought me back
from the eye clinic
had blocked the road outside our house
for half a minute)
and say to him,
'Can you think of a better way
I should be getting back from hospital?'

I do the shopping on my own.
Even handling the card machine
feels good.

Do I have an accounts book
that records my losses?
I see a ledger with
ear, eye, hair, and feeling in my toes
as outgoings.

On the street corner
I'm still proud I can plod with the shopping.
Old friends standing by their gates
ask me how I am.
I point at bits of me
and begin at each place with:
'I can't ... '
'I can't ... '
One says, 'Does the world
look different to you?'
I looked:
children cantering home
the sun splintering off car windows.
'Yes,' I said and thought
how sharp to suspect that's how
I think.

I walked the last stretch
feeling the pull of the shopping
on my arm.
I thought how accounts and ledgers
only notice gains and losses,
not differences.
Just as I've pushed myself
to get to M&S and back
couldn't I make an effort
to think I'm not a ledger?
I am what I've become?
And it never stops:
we are always becoming.

I have Alternate Days Syndrome.
The first day of Alternate Days Syndrome
I go shopping and lift 5kg weights.
The second day of Alternate Days Syndrome
I sit on the sofa
and doze with my eyes half-open.
The third day of Alternate Days Syndrome
I go shopping and lift 5kg weights.
The fourth day of Alternate Days Syndrome
I sit on the sofa
and doze with my eyes half-open.

You know the rest.

I play pinball pain.
A pain ball pings round my body
yesterday, my knee
– that clears
today, my ear
– it'll clear
last week, my toe
– it's cleared.
I'm Caliban
'pinched' by an invisible Prospero:
He tells me that he sends me
prickly sea urchins
in the 'vast of night'.

Caliban complains.
I tell myself not to.
Long before this
I invented a Mr Man book:
Mr Kvetch.
Whenever you meet him
he kvetches.
You talk to him about the trees
Mr Kvetch kvetches
about the pain in his back.
You talk about the taste of the soup

Mr Kvetch kvetches about his itchy legs.

Mr Kvetch is all kvetch.

Michael, don't be Mr Kvetch.

'kvetch': to moan or complain in Yiddish

People stop me in the park
and say they're glad
I'm up and about.
I guess it feels to them
as if I've postponed death,
fended it off for a bit longer.
I don't want to be the messenger
of false hope though.
I didn't cancel death.
It just didn't happen right then.
And it is what we all do.
Life is postponing death.
When I meet people
and they say
they're glad to see me
I tell them I'm not dead.

It's autumn
and I am becalmed
in a fear of winter cold
and the news comes in
that all that fever,
and this busy prickly virus
attaching itself to my cells
might not be a barricade
against it happening again.

Here, though,
I'm in the midst of beginnings:
you love, are starting a big, new thing
a change;
our daughter is buying lamps and
wooden spoons
before she leaves for university;
our son hovers on the edge
of a return to school,
GCSE worksheets lie open on the table;
and my granddaughter
not yet two years old
sits on the blanket outside:
we do
round and round the garden

like a teddy bear,
again and again and again,
she kicks a ball
and we all clap.

VIII.
THESE ARE THE HANDS

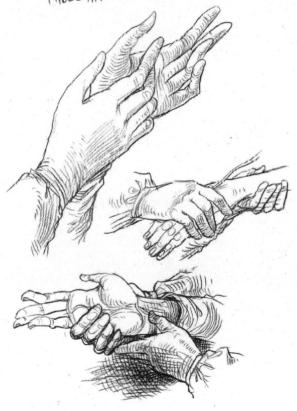

for the 60th anniversary of the NHS

These are the hands
That touch us first
Feel your head
Find the pulse
And make your bed.

These are the hands
That tap your back
Test the skin
Hold your arm
Wheel the bin

Change the bulb
Fix the drip
Pour the jug
Replace your hip.

These are the hands
That fill the bath
Mop the floor
Flick the switch
Soothe the sore

Burn the swabs
Give us a jab
Throw out sharps
Design the lab.

And these are the hands
That stop the leaks
Empty the pan
Wipe the pipes
Carry the can

Clamp the veins
Make the cast
Log the dose
And touch us last.

Michael has continued to write poems about his recovery since the initial release of *Many Different Kinds of Love*, published now for the first time in this paperback edition.

Every now and then
I get the memory of the hospital smell again.
A déjà-whiff.
I'm beginning to think
I'm attached to hospital now.
My head lives there.

If I could meet each and everyone
of you who cared for me
who cared for all that time,
I wouldn't know how to get through
everything I wanted to say
because I wouldn't know the words
to say what I thought,
and because I wouldn't be able to say
all the words that I wanted to say
because I get overcome thinking
of what you did for me.

If I could meet each and everyone
of you who cared for me
who cared for all that time,
I would try as hard as I could
to find the words
to say what I thought
and I would hope I could say
all the words that I wanted to say
and not get overcome thinking
of what you did for me

because I would like you to hear
what I think
because I would like you to know
what I think.

I meet Marjie
one of the nurses who looked after me
in intensive care
and wrote me a diary entry
in my Patient Diary book.

She sees me talking to the consultant
in the hospital garden.
Her face is delighted
but for a second
almost frightened.

I wonder in that second
if she thinks I'm a ghost.
I had put on such a good impression
of being dead.

I sit in the garden
and think of the story of the Unquiet Grave:
I'm wandering about dead
unable to be still
because Emma wouldn't let go of me.

When people say, 'It's good to see you,'
I'll tell them I'm a dybbuk -
a Jewish ghost.

'I'm an audiologist,' she said,
'have you heard of that?'

After 2 years of chemo
and an op that took away
half her jaw
my mother's body was wasted
and she stared at us from
one good eye
saddened and bewildered.
It was as if we had punished her.
My father took me to one side
and said he was having dreams
that she was in Belsen.

Days became days for learning:

A day
for learning to eat
A day
for learning to talk

A day
for learning to stand up.
A day
for learning to walk.

Days became days for walking:

A day
for walking round the house
A day
for walking out the house

A day
for walking to the corner.
A day
for walking round the corner.

Days become days for turning a corner.

The daily outpourings of News 24
are like water.
It flows over the crimes and disasters
of those who rule over us.
February and March
when they toyed with the idea
that hundreds of thousands of us should die,
have slipped from view.
New crimes, new disasters are waiting their turn.

I am the medical experiment
I am the politician's dream
I am the scientist's calculation
I am the journalist's headline

My eye is the collateral damage
My ear is the necessary wound
My blood clots are the inevitable consequence
My toes are the concomitant contribution

We are here to give you herd immunity
we are here to save your business
we are here to save the politicians' skins
we are here to say nothing

We are the dead
We are the long covids
We are the there-but-for-grace-of-god-go-you
We are you.

Worried today
that the last bit of sound
my left ear ekes out of the air,
was no longer available to me on that side.
That narrow band of megahertz
had finally gone.
Several hours of mild sadness.
Then – medical breakthrough:
I discovered
I hadn't switched my hearing-aid on.

I have been given names for
what I should be doing:
The Brace, the Diagonal Wood Chop
The Bridge, the Dead Bug,
The Bird Dog, the Plank.
As I do them, I say to myself,
'I'm doing the "Bird Dog",' and
It feels like I'm doing something
Important.

My hearing aid amplifies
the sound of me crunching
the seeds in dried figs.
I'm eating fireworks.

I've just watched a film of me
in intensive care.
I look dead.
My skin is grey,
My hair is limp,
My eyes stare at nothing.
Then a doctor comes to me
And asks me something.
I answer.
My eyes look frightened.

I have no memory of this conversation.
It's gone.

The camera has kept it.

I look at me.
Such a dry face.
Hospital gown.
Tubes.
I can see my father's last days there.

DREAM

I was in a place
where I couldn't see or hear.
I couldn't feel what I was touching
couldn't taste my tongue.
Now I'm back
I remember a field of bodies.

We stared with eyes
that couldn't see
but I had enough power in my arms
to pull me out from under
and by tugging on legs and heads
I got free.

I took a look back
and saw ten thousand elbows
hips and knees.
They belonged to people,
and I didn't know why
I wasn't one of them.

Today
I
will
wear
my
underpants
the
right
way
round.

For months
I've been saying to myself
I'm not strong enough
to climb Muswell Hill.
Then
I started to wonder if maybe
I could.
But I didn't dare.
I was worried that
I might get stuck halfway up.
So I didn't climb Muswell Hill.
It got bigger and steeper.
Beyond what I would be able to do.
Today
as it was getting dark
I took hold of the thought
that it was too big
and I walked down Muswell Hill
saying to myself,
every step down
will have to be a step up.
I popped in to see my son
who lives at the bottom of Muswell Hill
said goodbye
and then I went for it.

I started to climb Muswell Hill.

It's something like a 65 metre climb.

I said to myself

I mustn't stop.

Put one foot in front of the other

keep moving

one step

one step

one foot in front of each other.

A couple of times I touched the ivy

on a wall by my side:

but that's all.

No other help.

Today I climbed Muswell Hill.

Yesss!

I was bad.

I took a wrong turning in life:

I got old.

I didn't mean to.

Perhaps someone led me astray.

Perhaps I was weak.

I just got into bad ways:

and I kept doing it:

kept on and on being old.

So I got my punishment.

Fair dos.

I was caught.

Sentenced to death.

Part of herd immunity, they said.

But I got a reprieve

thanks to doctors and nurses

who seemed to think I shouldn't swing for it.

You never forget things like that.

I'll always be grateful to those people

who saw a bit of good in me

in spite of everything.

I'm glad I've been given a second chance.

I'm trying not to be old now.

But it's hard.

I get tempted.

I look in the mirror
and see wrinkles
and start to stay to myself,
'You're old.'
But you have to stop yourself
don't you?
Because being old is dangerous
when you're around people
who say your time's up,
you've got to go . . .

I've been trying to get away from
feeling precarious.
I do exercises:
squats, weights;
walking firmly
heels down first and hard.

I think it's a hoax.
I'm just trying to trick myself.
I'm play-acting at being who I was.

Beneath the surface
is Wobbly Man
who bumps into doors
and forgets which club Arsenal beat
last time Arsenal won the FA Cup.
It's not just that I look like
I'm walking on mud.
I'm thinking on mud.

Sorry to revisit this
but I can remember something else:
this is how I said it was . . .

"A doctor is standing by my bed
asking me if I would sign a piece of paper
which would allow them to put to sleep
and pump air into my lungs
'Will I wake up?'
'There's a 50:50 chance.'
'If I say no?' I say.
'Zero.'
And I sign."

The thing is
I can remember something else.
I remember thinking:

50:50?
That's pretty good.

Now that they've replaced my own lens
with a plastic one,
every day the view through my eyes is
different:
a new blur to my right
a brightened slash in the corner
and two trees where there was one yesterday.

At first
as I walked out of the hospital door
it was all seasons of mists
without much fruitfulness
but perhaps that was the sticking plaster
over the transparent eye patch
making it not transparent
and the other eye is always Clint Eastwood anyway
playing misty for me.

As Vik the surgeon
took out my own lens
he said, 'Fat.'
We had looked at it on the scan
and I imagined it between his fingers
like a button
(I once cut a sheep's lens in half
in Biology)

and he threw that bit of me
in a bin.
Unwanted spare part.

I stared at the arc lights

He called for a lens
and counted
1, 2, 3
as if it was going to leap from a petri dish
into the gaping hole of my eye.
I guessed he squeezed it in somehow.

I remembered drawing tiny muscles
thinning and thickening a lens.

I lay still, not daring to move
in case something missed.

And I wondered how those tiny muscles
connected to my new lens . . .
or will it be as I imagined it:
a button in my eye
as inert as a magnifying glass?

I was good at not moving,
though I gulped twice.

I should have asked to keep my lens.
I could have kept it in a jar of salt water.

What with all that Shakespeare in me
since I was ever,
I thought of that shout, 'Pluck out his eyes!'
and then: 'Out vile jelly!'
If I could see it on the mantlepiece
in its jar
I wouldn't think it vile.
I might think of it like
a stuffed favourite cat
in its glass case.

What a beautiful day!
Uh-huh! Vertigo!
Dizzy, whizzy Vertigo!
I can't go over it.
I can't go under it.
I've got to go through it.
Whirl-whirly! Whirl-whirly! Whirl-whirly!

I wake up in the night:
the room is spinning.
I look at the lamp hanging from the ceiling.
It's moving to the right
again and again
as if it's on runners.
Emma is asleep.
I think about waking her
to tell her
but what could she do?
I stare hard at the lamp
trying to hold it in its place
but it has a life of its own
moving and moving.
I close my eyes again
to stop myself seeing it.
Deep inside
the engine of my mind
is turning over so fast
that I can feel it in my temples.

I meet my grown-up children in the park.
They take the dad for a walk.
I don't have a lead,
I don't run off
and I don't sniff other dads.

I don't know them.

They were next to me in the ward.

We were in a coma

Side by side.

The 'Prof' said we were dying at a rate

of 42%.

If there were 20 of us, 8 died.

I don't know them.

I don't remember them.

Remember them.

Epitaph for Michael Rosen
He only ever ate one oyster.

An exclusive interview with Michael Rosen,
to mark the paperback publication of
Many Different Kinds of Love

You have written many very successful (and much-loved) books in your long career, but *Many Different Kinds of Love* was your first *Sunday Times* bestseller. What about the book do you think has resonated the most with readers?

It seems as if people have heard first-hand what incredible efforts, care, skill and love have been directed at someone who would have died. We came up with a way of telling this from several sides: from the point of view of the patient – me! ; the point of view of the nurses who we hear from directly through their letters; and the point of view of my wife, Emma, as she writes to the family and to me while the ups and downs of my illness unfold. This gives readers a 3D story, which makes it very much more than a sick person's story. It tells the story of an era.

There's another element that people have reacted to: how does someone deal with the fact that they know they nearly died and what does it feel like to recover from such a place? I tried to tell that in as direct and as an honest a way as possible, sometimes becoming very basic and visceral, because that's where you get to sometimes: just you, in your body, with your body. I think that has surprised some people.

Could you tell us more about the process of writing the book? Was it a cathartic experience exploring such a challenging time, and did you find you gained more insight into your illness by writing about it?

I write because I want to write. I started after I came home, jotting things down, trying to explore and understand what had happened to me. At that point, that's all it was: sorting it. The way I do it is to dive in with words rather than sentences, or sometimes an opening phrase that I've said to myself as I'm waking up in the morning. Then, I don't think in paragraphs or chapters. I think in lines. So I write a line and when the next thought or word or phrase comes to me, I start the next line. I have a sense that I'm unfolding something on to the page and each new line comes where the crease of the fold is. I unfold each line. I try to not to froth or over-emotionalise about things. Mostly I want the 'I' of the poem (me!) to be a witness who is a bit amazed, bemused, naively trying to follow what's happening, occasionally amused but also a bit reserved. I don't want to let on very often what I am actually feeling. I realise that that is almost the opposite of what we think poetry is for but there are poetic traditions that are less like the English lyric tradition of pouring out an emotion: ancient Chinese poetry, the 'imagist' poetry of the first modernists, or the detached writing of someone like Raymond Carver. That's what I'm trying to do.

Is it cathartic? You bet! It's a prop for me. I think of the page as a friend who I can talk to: someone who doesn't mock or sneer at me or flatter me. It just receives and accepts.

The insights come so long as I am truthful about what things look, sound and feel like. If I cheat, it's just a waste of time. All the poems that are in the book feel truthful to me. I chucked away the untruthful ones.

The nurses' diaries are at the heart of the book, and perform a vital service in telling us what was happening when you were in a coma. When you read the diaries, was there anything that struck or surprised you?

I'm not ducking the question when I say everything surprised me. They are overwhelming in their kindness and care. Every word! I love the way that they tell me who they are, what they usually do, like whether they've been drafted in from other part of the hospital or something to do with their children. It really is very humbling to think that someone who is, let's say, a physiotherapist, has come over to the intensive care ward and is dealing with this unconscious lump in a bed. I love their details: how they explain to me for example that they have to shave me in case my beard infects the tracheostomy wound, or that one supports Derby while I support Arsenal. And I love how they urge me to get better, right from the start, not knowing then that I would be sedated for 40 days.

There is a power in their writing that comes from them doing a job, telling me what's being going on in the ward and what they've done. They have a direction, which is on the cover of the 'Patient Diary': 'The diary may help with the patient's post-Critical Care recovery by providing them with information and insight into a time when they were not aware'. Everything they wrote does exactly this – it helps me and gives me insight into a time when I was not aware. These letters prove to me over and over again that there is something beautiful about writing for such a purpose. I remember every day that people who wrote these letters saved my life. They tell me that they stood round my bed and sang me 'Happy Birthday' when I was just an inert blob. It's incredible.

The book is one of the first published accounts of Long Covid and shows the twists and turns of recovering from a severe illness, particularly how it can transform one's sense of identity. Has your experience changed your perspective on life?

I think so. At one point in the book, I say that I have learnt how to own my own frailty. I might change that a bit and say that I have learnt how to own my fragility – or at least I'm trying to. I often feel as if I am easily broken. It's not that I thought I was superman before I got ill, but I think I may have been arrogant enough to have thought that I was in pretty good nick, all things considered. Now I think of myself as a veteran carrying wounds from some kind of major event, like an earthquake.

I have to work hard on the matter of thinking of the two kinds of 'me': the one before and the one since. It's easy to mourn the loss of the one before, to feel that it has died. Or, alternatively, to think of the one since as unworthy or incomplete. I have to work hard to not think this. That takes time and effort, some of it mental and the other physical – lifting weights, doing exercises, walking purposefully (!).

At the time of doing these things, it's all very short of laughs. I'm someone who had always very much enjoyed finding the absurdities and jokes of everyday life. I hope that all this stuff that I keep describing as 'work' isn't killing the gags. I'm always very glad when I find something comical in the gruesome.

In writing about the pandemic, it's almost impossible to avoid writing about the political aspect of Covid-19, and this is something *Many Different Kinds of Love* discusses in detail. How do you balance the political and the personal in your work?

I think this illness is political. As I say in the book, I slowly came to realise that the government made (or did not make) crucial decisions in February and March 2020. Whatever they had done in that time would have affected all our lives. I think they took the wrong decisions and then made a right decision too late. That view, though, is not me turning the illness (which happened to me personally) into something political. As I say, if they had taken what I would now regard as the right decisions, that would still be political. The World Health Organisation talk of 'public health policies'. Again, all health policies are public and political, and hurrah for that. Governments should be there working out the best way to protect us and help us.

I am grateful and delighted that the book gives voice to what is the best of the NHS, people of many different backgrounds using their skills, knowledge and training to help people, care for them and go beyond care to another place that feels to me like love. And yes, though this is utterly personal, it's also utterly political in that it has to be arranged, organised and worked for so that it can happen.

You'll be continuing to explore the theme of recovery in a forthcoming book, *Getting Better*. What can readers expect to find in that, and is it a continuation of the journey we find you on in *Many Different Kinds of Love*?

As I started to think about 'recovery', I found myself thinking over what other things have I had to recover from in my life. In one of my reveries, I went through things like the time I was knocked down in the road and was in hospital for 10 weeks; the time my brother and I discovered that we had had a brother who died; the death of my son Eddie; the family blank about the relatives who had been killed in the Holocaust. And then what about the more minor setbacks, humiliations and 'downs'? Times when I felt that I was stuck or had failed my parents as when I knew that I couldn't go on studying Medicine (ok, I know the irony of that one now!). As I thought about all these and more, I started to wonder if there's a model of us as human beings that is as though we are all recoverers. At some point – or at many points in our lives – we have to try to recover. In biology there is a process called 'homeostasis', which describes how organisms have means to restore themselves to equilibrium with the circumstances they are in. I am thinking about how this is what I've been doing with the trials and crises of my life ...

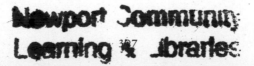